19. APR 99
02. SEP 99
23. OCT 99
16 MAY 00
01
12 FEB 02
12 JUL 04

CL69100K

I LOOKED IN THE MIRROR AND SCREAMED

I LOOKED IN THE MIRROR AND SCREAMED

Healthier Eating for Teenagers

DR LINDA OJEDA

Piccadilly Press • London

Copyright © Linda Ojeda, 1993

First published in Great Britain by Piccadilly Press, 1994
First published in the USA by Hunter House Inc
2200 Central Avenue, Suite 202, Alameda, CA 94501 as
Safe Dieting for Teens

All rights reserved. No part of this publication may be
reproduced, stored in a retrieval system or transmitted,
in any form, or by any means electronic, mechanical,
photocopying, recording or otherwise without prior
permission of the copyright owner.

The right of Linda Ojeda to be identified as Author of this
work has been asserted by her in accordance with the
Copyright, Designs and Patents Act 1988.

Typeset by Textype Typesetters
Printed and bound by Biddles Ltd., Guildford
for the publishers, Piccadilly Press Ltd.,
5 Castle Road, London NW1 8PR

A catalogue record for this book is available
from the British Library

ISBN: 1 85340 214 1 (trade paperback)
1 85340 209 5 (hardback)

Linda Ojeda PhD is American. She is an author and
lecturer on nutrition, dieting, and exercise and is a
qualified nutritional consultant. She has written two
other books *Menopause Without Medicine* and
Exclusively Female which is a nutritional approach to
PMS and other menstrual disorders.

To my children, who are no longer teenagers, Jill and Joey

Important Notice

The material in this book is intended to provide a review of Dr Ojeda's recommendations for safe and effective teenage weight loss. Every effort has been made to provide accurate and dependable information. However, health care professionals have differing opinions, and advances in medical and scientific research are made very quickly, so that some of the information may become outdated.

Therefore, the publisher, author, editors and professionals quoted in the book cannot be held responsible for any error, omission, or dated material. They cannot be held responsible for the endorsement of any outside weight loss agency. Any of the recommendations described within should be tried only under the guidance of a licensed health-care practitioner. The author and publisher assume no responsibility for any outcome of the use of this programme of weight loss in self-treatment or under the care of a licensed practitioner.

If you have a question concerning your health, weight loss, or the appropriateness or application of the programme described in this book, consult your health-care professional.

This book has been read by a UK nutritionist.

Table of Contents

Introduction xi

Chapter 1: Are You Really Overweight?.... 1–9
Appraising the Situation 2
How Did That Fat Find Your Body? 4

Chapter 2: Girls' Special Diet Dilemma... 11–19
Girls Are Born With More Fat Than Boys 12
Girls Make Fat Easily. 12
Female Hormones and Cravings 15
Female Hormones and Weight Loss 16
The Pill and Weight Gain 17
Inability to Handle Carbohydrates 18
Tradition 18

Chapter 3: Eating Disorders 21–31
Anorexia 21
Bulimia. 25
Compulsive Eating 27

Chapter 4: How *Not* to Diet 33–39
Very Low Calorie Fad Diets 34
Skipping Meals 35
Commercial Programmes. 36
Liquid Diets 36
Pills and Diet Aids 37

Chapter 5: Dieting Starts in the Mind, Not the Mouth ... 41–52
- How Do You Feel About Being Overweight? 42
- Feeling Good About Yourself 45
- Why I Want to Lose Weight.................. 47
- Design Your Dreams........................ 49

Chapter 6: Exercise and Physical Activity 53–62
- Why Exercise? 54
- Aerobic Exercise 57

Chapter 7: Designing Your Own Diet ... 63–82
- Plan of Action 64
- What Do You Eat Now? 67
- Getting Rid of Fat Promoters................ 70
- Snack Attacks 75
- Healthy Eating Keeps You Slim 79
- Fine-Tuning Your Plan 81

Chapter 8: Eating Out.................. 83–89
- Restaurant Food Guide...................... 84
- Surviving Fast-Food Joints 85
- Tips for Success 87

Appendix A: Calories in Common Foods..... 91

Appendix B: Resources: Where to Get More Help 103

Introduction

This book is written for teenagers who want to lose 5 or 50 pounds. Even though I don't like the word "diet", I use it because it is the word that we associate with weight loss. But let's face it: most diets don't work. They are short-term answers to a long-term problem. They deprive you of foods you like and they make you hungry, not to mention a little crazy. Many of them are unhealthy and unsafe. And almost always, the weight you've lost comes right back the minute you stop "dieting".

So, why have I written a diet book for teenagers? Simple: to tell you that diets are not effective in keeping weight off, and more important, to save you the time, money, and heartache that we older dieters have suffered from trying all the new diet gimmicks that crop up each year.

The idea for writing this diet book came to me while I was working for some of the top weight-loss programmes. I saw my clients regain their weight after being off the programme a while, and I heard their discouraging and frustrating stories. It was obvious that these structured diets lacked something. So I began working with many of these so-called failures, and together we tried to work out how they could keep their weight off. We found out that the closer the "weight-loss" diet was to a real, everyday diet, the easier it was to follow and maintain.

Every diet I helped design for these clients was different, because every person has different tastes and eating habits, social life, work schedule, and interests. I think this may have been why teenagers were especially unsuccessful in the structured programmes. They wanted variety, but the counsellors yelled every time they creatively altered the established rules. Even though the teenagers substituted healthier foods, it wasn't in the company's rules to deviate. That would mean that people would not buy the prepared foods they were told to buy, and the company would lose all that money. Commercial weight-loss programmes teach you to be dependent on them, so when you gain your weight back you will return and buy another programme.

The latest research on dieting shows one thing clearly. Structured programmes and crash diets do not work. What does work is a plan that is based on LOWERING CALORIES and INCREASING ACTIVITY. The diet you follow to lose weight should be very close to the diet you are going to stay on for the rest of your life. Think about all the diet plans you know. How many of them could you live with forever? How long can you last on apples and Diet Coke? How many weeks until you become sick at the thought of opening up another boxed diet delight? Boring diets don't last long.

Many programmes that promise you will lose several pounds a week are ineffective and even harmful for both physical and psychological reasons. Extremely low calorie diets (less than 1,000 calories per day) create a condition in the body that lowers the metabolism, so that when the dieter returns to normal eating, she or he gains weight very quickly. Something else that is discouraging, which few people know, is that a very low-calorie diet can lead to uncontrollable eating or bingeing. I think that these nutritionally poor diets made popular by our obsession with thinness may be creating the epidemic of eating disorders that we are witnessing.

So, the plan in this book is not a real "diet". It will not tell you what to eat or provide you with a list of "good" foods and "bad" foods. I don't believe foods should be categorized as ones we can eat (carrots and cottage cheese) and ones we can't (chocolate cake and doughnuts). We all know what happens when we're told we *can't* have something! The forbidden food just keeps calling our name until the last crumb has been devoured. I also don't like connecting guilty feelings to one of my favourite pastimes. It takes away the pleasure of eating, and that's a shame. Eating is fun; we should enjoy the experience.

You must be thinking you picked up the wrong book! Yes, this is a weight-loss book, and I'm telling you food is not your enemy. In fact, nothing is out of bounds. If a chocolate doughnut is the only thing that is going to satisfy you today, go for it. You know you will anyway. So, eat it slowly, and enjoy each and every bite.

What this book is all about is CHOICE. Losing weight is not a mystery. You have to lower your calorie intake, burn calories through exercise, or both. These are the options. However, there are many ways to accomplish this and you have to decide what works for you. For example, you can cut down on the amount of food you eat, you can substitute foods that have less fat in them, or you can space your meals, which raises your metabolic rate. The trick is, YOU decide what route to take (not me or any other expert), because what YOU choose, you will follow. This is your diet. You design it so that you're happy with it and successful.

Since making good choices is the key to success for any diet, you need to know exactly what you are doing now in terms of what you eat and your levels of physical activity. Certain lifestyles make dieting easier, others make it harder. Some habits are easy to change, others are nearly impossible. It will be up to you to decide which habits you want to alter and which ones you will accept. Once this is understood, you can start making realistic plans to change some of your behaviour. You won't have to change your life totally like you do when you start a "diet". And, you can take it slowly and get used to making one change at a time. This is the easiest, most effective way to lose weight.

I do not promise that you will be slim and trim by Saturday night—or even *next* Saturday night. What I do guarantee is that if you hang in there and follow the principles I give you, you will lose your weight safely and you will also keep it off.

I'm sure you want to know how you can lose pounds quickly, but try to be patient. It didn't take you two months to put the weight on, and it won't take just a few weeks to take if off. As you start this programme, think about it as something you are going to work at for a while. Think of it as learning a new skill, like playing tennis or the piano. Once you've been taught the fundamentals, all you have to do is practise. At first it seems awkward and difficult, but after a while it comes easily. Controlling your weight won't always be the struggle it is today. Really.

Here's a fundamental weight-loss fact to remember. Do you have any idea how many calories it takes to lose a pound of fat? Go ahead, guess. It takes 3,500 calories to *make* a pound of fat, so the reverse is true—**to lose one pound, you have to cut out or burn off 3,500 calories.** There are a number of ways to do this. I'll give you some alternatives and then you can take it from there and think up some of your own.

Did you know that how you feel about yourself and your reasons for wanting to change your body are just as important as counting calories? If you don't like who you are, you're not likely to do anything positive about improving how you look. I'd like to help you lose some pounds if that is what you want. More important, I hope to get you to think about your many great qualities and be happy with them. Don't feel you have to look and be like anyone else. In fact, isn't it more fun being a little different? Like yourself as you are today and then if there are things you want to work on, go for it. But do it for *yourself*, because it's what *you* want, not for any other reason.

As you can tell, this is not your typical diet. And because it's not, it will work. If you want to keep the fat off permanently, then you are going to have to change some things in your life. You don't have to change every "bad" habit. You will know by your weight loss what is enough, and I think you will be surprised that you can still get away with some things you thought you had to give up forever.

Small changes can make a big difference in your body. If you leave one tablespoon of butter off your morning toast (that's 100 calories), in one year you will lose 10 pounds. That's just eliminating a single item from your diet. Everything else stays the same. Think about this: if you exercised away 300 extra calories a day, four times a week, you could lose 16 pounds a year. Doing both equals 26 pounds lost in one year. Get the picture? Small yet consistent changes will take your fat off forever. Those are great results.

I don't want to make this sound TOO easy! You are going to have to work at this plan. Any real change in life takes time and effort. This book is all about you and what you want out of life. Please use this book—write in it, make it your own private diary for self-improvement. Make the effort. You know you're worth it!

1
Are You Really Overweight?

So you think you're fat. Or maybe not "fat" fat—you just want to lose a little weight. I want to ask: why? Who told you you were fat? How do you know? Does your mother nag you every time you put something in your mouth? Do friends call you "Chubs"? Do strangers give you that she-would-be-so-pretty-if-she-lost-weight look? Or do you just FEEL overweight? Your best friend wears clothes two sizes smaller than you. You feel really gross when you go shopping with her. Thumbing through magazines is depressing too. The models are so perfect and so thin, not one normal-looking female in the bunch.

I don't know many people who are totally comfortable with their looks. It seems most of us want to look like someone else. We compare our bodies, clothes, and hairstyles to friends, film stars, singers, and athletes. Whatever look is in today is what we want. I remember when we all wanted to look like super skinny model Twiggy. Some of my more full-figured friends at that time actually tied down their boobs to look more like her. This was before your time, but it shows the extent to which we will go to look "in". Really!

You are all probably more likely to remember George Michael, or Madonna. What a dynamic impact she has had. At one time half the young girls on the street seemed to be wearing lace underwear on the outside as well as the inside.

We are all influenced by people we admire, and it's

not necessarily bad either. It's quite natural to want to dress and look like those we find attractive. That is, unless we carry it too far and forget that we too have our own personality, and a special originality.

Are you uncomfortable with your mirror image? What do you feel you need: a new hairstyle, the right makeup, pretty fingernails, someone to show you how to dress? If you don't know what you want, talk to someone who can help you bring out your best qualities. Too often we concentrate on what's WRONG with us rather than what's RIGHT. Do you know what your good points are? List them. Are you stuck? Ask your very best friend, your mum, sister, brother or cousin. Anyone who will be honest, yet kind.

I don't think you should get hung up on your looks. Nothing is more boring than people who constantly gawk at themselves in the mirror. On the other hand, when we look as good as we can, we feel better about ourselves and then the whole world looks brighter. So, once you have made that positive step to improve your image, feel good about it and move on to other things. Stop comparing your thighs to the skinniest girl in the class and your nose to a supermodel's. Be proud of your individuality and your uniqueness.

I assume you are reading this book because the first thing you want to work on is your weight. That's great. I know when you feel fat you often feel unattractive and generally bad about yourself. But I would like to suggest that you don't wait until you have lost weight to enhance your appearance in other areas. Start appreciating yourself and doing things for yourself as you are right now.

*A*PPRAISING THE SITUATION

Before you even think of dieting, ask yourself some basic questions. Such as, do I really need to lose weight?

Am I sure? The answer might be YES if:

1. Your doctor tells you you would be healthier if you did.
2. Your parents think it's necessary.
3. School teachers have made comments jokingly.
4. Your friends make fun of you.

On the other hand, the answer might be NO if:

1. Your parents and friends tell you that you don't need to lose weight, even though you see a fat person in the mirror.
2. You are under the normal weight for your age.
3. Your doctor insists that it would be unhealthy for you to lose weight.
4. Your only reason to lose weight is because your thighs or hips are not as small as your friends' (this is not a weight problem but is due to body structure).

If you have decided that you definitely need to shed some pounds, how many do you think will put you at your ideal weight? Most people have a number in mind. They want to weigh 8 stone, or 9 stone, or whatever. Sometimes we want to weigh the same as our best friend. The number shouldn't be that important, as long as it's not unrealistic for us. It's great to have a goal in mind. Just consider that it is open for change. If you get to where you look and feel good but you're still not 8 stone, forget the number.

Another suggestion before you start—don't get too hung up on daily numbers. I mean the numbers on the scales. In fact, don't weigh yourself more than once a week. Personally, I think even that is too often. Scales do not always reflect fat loss. What we weigh at any particular time depends on our hormonal balance, what we had for supper last night, or how much liquid we are holding, and the scales may not show a fat loss when there might actually be one. I think it is a bad idea psychologically, too. If you weigh less, you celebrate with pizza, and if you weigh more, you drown your sorrows in ice-cream. Let's face it, this is a no-win situation. Stay away from the scales until your trousers get baggy. Once you're at your goal, don't be fanatical with the scales either. RELAX, and enjoy your success!

How did that fat find your body?

Some people say the simple reason for excess flab is that you eat too much or you don't exercise enough. If this is true, then why can your friend devour two Big Macs, a large fries, chocolate milkshake and an apple turnover while you have to stick with a plain hamburger and a Diet Coke? She doesn't have an inch to pinch and you're saddled with serious thighs.

There really is more to this weight loss thing than calories and exercise. Being overweight is a complex condition that is caused by several factors: heredity, individual body metabolism, emotional environment, food choices, and inactivity.

Heredity

There is no doubt that you inherit the tendency to be either fat or thin from your mum and dad. The facts are that if one parent is overweight there is a 40% chance that you will be too. If both parents are overweight, your chances double to 80%. But if you are reading this and looking at pudgy parents, don't throw up your hands in dismay. There is still hope. You are not doomed to wearing baggy trousers and oversized shirts forever. There is no question that those family genes may be waiting to get you, but there are other possibilities. Consider what your parents eat and drink daily. Do they eat mostly fatty foods, like steak, sausage, bacon, biscuits, chips, and dips? Do they eat large amounts of food at one time and have second and third helpings? Do they drink alcohol several nights a week? Do they snack on ice cream and cake before going to bed? Are they couch potatoes? Do they drive rather than walk – even if they're going a short distance? These habits can also be the culprits, not just the genes.

Individual body metabolism

The way the body makes and burns fat is complicated. One thing we do know is that bodies don't all react the same way. Some people store fat more easily (most women) and some burn calories at a faster rate (most men). You see this all the time. You go out with friends who eat everything in sight and don't gain an ounce, while you smell the doughnuts and watch your hips expand. This unfair fact of life is due to metabolic differences. While we may never be like those lucky few, however, we can make some changes in our lifestyle that will help to speed up our metabolism.

Your physical structure provides a clue to whether you are likely to gain weight easily. The short, stocky build generally is the one that gains pounds fastest. The shorter the person, the fewer calories required to maintain weight. If you are short and you eat like your friend who is tall, watch out. It will catch up with you.

The tall, slender, beanpole types rarely have a problem with too much fat. All of us who constantly struggle with flab hate these people for being able to enjoy so much food. If it is any consolation, though, skinny does not necessarily mean healthy. And we all want to be fit and healthy too, right?

Another characteristic we are born with is our appetite. While some people pick and nibble all day, others require three full meals to feel satisfied. When planning your daily diet, it is important to stay close to your natural inclinations as much as possible. Otherwise you may get totally frustrated and go bananas. If you require a lot of food at one time, there are tricks you can use to eat the quantity you need without getting too many calories. For example, have a bowl of soup or a piece of fruit half an hour before your meal, eat more slowly, and include more high fibre foods (fresh fruits and vegetables, whole grain breads and pasta) in your meal. They will fill you up but not out.

Emotional environment

Scientists do not agree on which is more responsible for causing people to be overweight—heredity or environment. Since they both play major roles, it really doesn't matter which one wins the debate. Now you know that you were born with a certain metabolism and there is little you can do about that. But what about your environment? Do you have any control? Up to a certain age, no. As you were growing up, your mum, dad, or someone else prepared the meals, bought the food, handed out goodies as she or he felt appropriate, and basically gave or denied you food. If your diet was reasonably varied and well-balanced and snacks were kept to a minimum, it's more than likely you will be of normal weight and size. However, if your parents preferred mostly high-fat foods, allowed you unlimited desserts, chips, sweets, and so on, and if they did not encourage you to exercise, you almost had no choice but to be an overweight child.

If the person who raised you used food to reward or punish you, it may show up now in your attitude towards food and eating. Do you remember being promised an ice-cream cone if you didn't tease your little sister or run through the racks of clothes in the shops? How about being denied your cake because you gave your peas to the dog? Sounds familiar? I'm embarrassed to admit that I used some of these tactics on my children when they were young. Don't be too critical of mum if she resorted to bribery. None of us is perfect. What I want you to ask yourself is, do you do this to yourself now? When you have finished a hard task, done well in the maths test, or just had a good day, do you celebrate with a special dinner or an extra dessert? How about if your day was the pits or just dull? Do you make yourself feel better by getting a pizza? I'll talk more about this later, but think about when and why you eat or overeat.

Habits may also be copied from friends or started for no reason at all. Sometimes teenagers (and adults) turn to food for comfort when there is friction at home. Any family situation which causes unhappiness or frustration may lead to overeating. Food can easily be the "cure" for loneliness, boredom, or anger. Unfortunately, once the food has been devoured, the problems are still there, as well as the guilt feelings for pigging out.

The life of a teenager seems to be non-stop stress. Look at some of the problems you have to face: school, grades, relationships (peers and parents), divorce, drugs, alcohol, acne, AIDS, the environment, nuclear bombs, and your future. I hope I didn't depress you. The point is, with all these stresses, who has time to worry about dieting? Trying not to freak out may be the best you can do. If you have a serious problem, family or other, please talk to someone you respect—a school teacher or counsellor, your vicar, or another member of your family. Just get help. If you are also overweight, don't worry so much about the weight yet. Working on one problem at a time is enough. Getting your emotional situation together is really the first and most important step in controlling your weight, as well as your life.

Food choices

Your parents decided what you ate up to a certain age. Now you have your own ideas. In counselling teenagers, I have found standard preferences: hamburgers, french fries, pizza, crisps, nachos, ice-cream, sweets, and chocolate. Am I close? You may like other food as well, but these seem to make the Top Ten. You may not know this about these favourites, but many of these are potential disasters for adding fat to the body. Not only are they high in calories, they are high in FAT calories—the worst kind.

Fat makes you fat. Fat calories are stored in the body quickly, much more easily than protein or starch calories. Therefore, when you make choices about where to cut down the calories, the best place to start is with high-fat foods. They're easy to spot. Foods that are high in fat are also high in calories.

I am not suggesting that you eliminate all these foods from your diet. You wouldn't anyway, would you? You can still go to McDonald's with your friends and order pizza at home. But when you do, be aware of the choices that are highest and lowest in fat calories.

Activity level

If there is one magic way to lose fat, it is increasing your general activity level by moving around more and exercising regularly. If you had to choose between cutting down on your calories or exercising, I would say start exercising first. People who just watch their calories and don't exercise usually regain their weight quickly once they start eating normally again. This happens because low-calorie dieting alone results in a loss of muscle mass and a lower metabolism. As soon as you eat the way you did before the diet, the weight creeps back.

Exercise, on the other hand, speeds up the metabolism and weight loss. I tell all my weight-loss classes that the basic reason why I exercise is so I can eat more! Yes, I like the fact that I feel better mentally and physically. I like the fact that exercise reduces stress and makes me healthy, but the real motivation for jogging and going to aerobics is so I can enjoy my cake.

I know many of you hate P.E. and despise sweating. I certainly did. But there are so many fun kinds of exercise outside school. Maybe you just haven't tried enough different ones to find the exercise you like. Even walking is great. It doesn't cost anything, and you don't have to go anywhere special to do it. Some teenagers have told me they are embarrassed to be seen in a leotard. Fine, with walking you can wear leggings or jeans. Another suggestion—how about getting an exercise video? There are all kinds, for all levels. I suggest that you rent one first before you decide to buy. Make sure that it is something you like and would do often.

In addition to regular exercise, just moving your body more every day burns additional calories. Create steps even when you don't have to. Take the stairs instead of the lift, use your feet instead of wheels, get on your bike rather than drive. These little extras can take off half a pound a week. So move it—and lose it!

2
Girls' Special Diet Dilemma

I don't know about you, but as I was growing up there were many things I didn't understand—and was afraid to ask about. Maybe that was more typical of my generation than yours. We didn't talk openly about things like sex, pregnancy, and contraception. In fact, we rarely even mentioned our periods to our best friends. Can you imagine that? The female body was a taboo topic. I'm so glad things have changed and girls are now free to discuss these subjects. The teenage years are scary enough. When you don't know what's going on and you don't feel comfortable asking, all sorts of strange thoughts go through your mind, exaggerating any problem.

Even though communication has improved over the years, there are some subjects that are not written about as much as others. This is true in the area of dieting and the female body. While dieting in general is a hot topic, the differences between males and females are often overlooked.

Female weight loss is affected by more variables than male weight loss. It is really true that girls gain weight more easily than guys, and shed pounds more slowly. It is also true that some girls have it easier than others, and even for the same individual, losing fat may be more difficult at certain times of the month than at others. Let's consider these points in more detail, one at a time.

GIRLS ARE BORN WITH MORE FAT THAN BOYS

The female body is different from the male. You've probably already noticed that. Our bodies are constructed to carry and feed an infant, regardless of whether or not we are having one. From the beginning of our childbearing years (menarche) to their completion (menopause), our body's composition and our female hormones continuously prepare us to carry on life. This basic difference, as wonderful and miraculous as it is, makes it easier for us to put on weight and harder for us to lose it.

From the day a baby girl comes into the world, she is at a disadvantage in terms of fat. The female body has almost twice as much fat as the male. While guys carry around more muscle (which burns calories), girls store more fat (which doesn't burn calories). Muscle tissue burns five calories per pound more than fat tissue. This means that if you ate the same foods as your boyfriend or brother, and he stayed the same, you would gain weight. On the other hand, if you maintained your weight eating the same food, he would lose it. Never diet with a male friend. It's too depressing!

As you read the exercise chapter, you will see that when girls exercise and increase their muscle mass, they too burn more calories, just like the guys. This doesn't mean the body becomes masculine—it can't, because female hormones prevent that. But it is a definite advantage for girls to build up their muscle and raise their metabolism. You will lose weight more quickly and you will be able to eat more.

GIRLS MAKE FAT EASILY

The female body has a high percentage of slow-burning fat tissue. And, even though most of us are not thrilled with this fact, it helps us to understand why our bodies fight us when we try to diet. As I mentioned before, our extra fat is necessary to survival and our body hates to lose it. In fact, our fat is so linked to child-bearing that when a female's body fat falls below 17% of her total weight, she will stop having periods and will no longer be able to carry a child. Our sex is designed for motherhood, whether we like it or not.

You probably know girls who stopped having periods when they got very skinny, or you may have friends who have not even started menstruating yet. Look at their bodies. You will see they don't have much body fat. When they put on some pounds, they will start or restart their cycle.

Oestrogen is the female hormone that directly affects shape and fat distribution. The more oestrogen your body makes, the more "full-figured" you are. In other words, you have more fat on your hips, thighs, and breasts. Some people refer to this as an hourglass figure. The good news is, this look is supposedly coming back, and I personally know many guys like it. The bad news is, this shape makes it easier for you to gain weight and harder for you to lose it.

Let me tell you more about oestrogen. As you probably know it is made in the ovaries. It is a hormone that loves to take the food you eat and turn it into fat. Remember, the female body is designed to keep fat on the body and it is oestrogen's job to make sure this happens. So, if your body naturally makes more oestrogen, your chances of being overweight are greater. But this is only part of the story. What you may not know is that oestrogen is also manufactured from fat. Therefore, if you have more fat on your body, you are also going to *make* more oestrogen.

So, here's the picture. The more oestrogen you have, the easier it is to store fat; the more fat you have, the more oestrogen you make. You can see that once you start gaining weight, the body becomes a virtual fat-making machine.

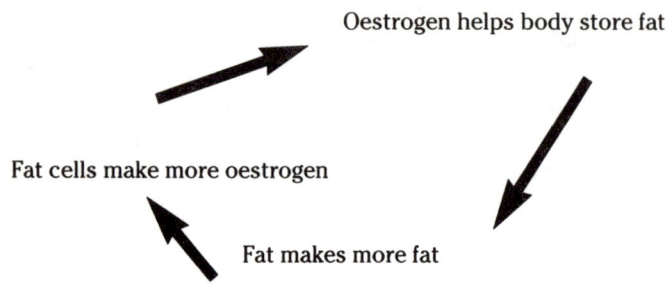

Now you can see why it is harder for females who naturally make more oestrogen to lose weight. Their bodies are working against them. While they struggle to lose fat, their bodies just love to make it. We often blame failure at dieting on our lack of will-power or self-control, when in fact it is our physiology. But don't take this knowledge and give up, thinking it's no use. You *can* lose the extra fat and you can keep it off. But you do have to work harder than a bloke and harder than your friend who was born to be a stick.

Let me give you a few tips that are especially important if you have a full-figured body:

1. **Watch high fat foods**, because fatty foods are stored faster than any other kind.
2. **Eat more high fibre foods** (fruits, vegetables, whole grain breads, cereals, and pastas), because they help to lower oestrogen levels in the body and assist in removing fat.
3. **Eat small meals more often**, since too much food at one time turns to fat.
4. **Watch salty foods**, because they retain water.
5. **Exercise regularly** to burn fat and build muscle.

Female Hormones and Cravings

A female's appetite appears to fluctuate with the ups and downs of her female hormones, oestrogen and progesterone. Oestrogen seems to reduce hunger while progesterone stimulates the appetite. After ovulation, which is halfway through the menstrual cycle (for most girls this is two weeks after your period), oestrogen levels fall and progesterone levels rise. When this happens, you may want to eat more than normal and you may find you crave particular foods like chocolate or crisps.

How many of you have powerful cravings for crisps, chocolate, biscuits, cheese puffs, or cake? I know there have been many days when I would make a special trip to the nearest bakery or finish off the stale potato crisps because of this driving desire. I have one friend who told me that in one day she ate a pound of sweets, a hot fudge sundae, and a chocolate mousse. I bet you can come up with a few stories of your own.

Food cravings can be caused by any number of things. It seems for many of us they get particularly strong right before our periods. Have you noticed this? If you haven't made that connection, the next time you want to eat everything in the kitchen, think about when your period is due. Chances are it's due in a few days.

Other things can also cause you to raid the refrigerator. Being overweight can itself result in binges, due to both psychological reasons (who cares? what's the use? food makes me feel good) and physical or hormonal causes (blood sugar imbalances, insulin response). Still other possibilities include a lack of certain vitamins and minerals and poor eating habits (like too much sugar). Which of these apply to you? It could be more than one. Look at the chart on pages 16–17 for ideas on how to deal with these cravings.

Female hormones and weight loss

In the second half of the menstrual cycle, when progesterone is more dominant, there are other physiological changes that tend to make dieting harder or downright impossible. Some girls retain extra water so they feel bloated and fat, their fingers and stomach swell, and their breasts are painful or sensitive. Maybe you have noticed that the week before your period you often weigh several pounds more than you expect. Don't worry. This is common. It just means you've gained water—not fat.

Retaining water is very discouraging to a dieter. You feel you've watched your calories all week and then you don't see the results on the scale. Even if you tell yourself it's probably water, psychologically you want to give up and give in. To avoid this, just before your period, when this is more likely to happen, relax on your diet. Don't expect to cut back on your calories. Concentrate on simply maintaining your weight, and look forward to going back to your diet in a few days.

If you are prone to water retention there are several practical things you can do to keep it under control. Watch the amount of salty and sugary food you eat, drink plenty of water (at least eight glasses a day), and eat several small meals rather than two or three large meals.

Controlling cravings

Hormonal—Sometimes just changing your diet can help with hormonal cravings. If you are eating three meals a day and you cut down on fat and sugar throughout the month, these cravings won't be as strong. If they are, you may need to talk to a nutritionist. Exercise may also help.

Overweight—Losing weight often helps with cravings. I won't say that they will be gone forever, but they may not be as bad when you reach your ideal weight.

Vitamin and mineral deficiencies—This may happen if your diet is poor. That means, you don't eat a variety of food, you eat food that has little nutritional value, or you don't eat enough calories. Changing these habits would make a big difference, but if you refuse to change, taking a vitamin/mineral supplement will help. No, it won't make up for the other things, but it might help.

Other hormones—Other hormones like insulin may cause cravings. If you eat a lot of sugar, the insulin response may make you crave even more sugar. If you starve yourself or go a day without eating, the same insulin response may cause you to overeat. If you pig out, a similar reaction may cause a craving. The way to prevent this insulin response is obvious—don't do these things.

Psychological responses—Some of the reasons we overeat are emotional. We substitute eating for feelings. This is really a harder problem to work out. If you overeat because you are bored, feel unloved, or are anxious about something, you need to deal with that issue first.

THE PILL AND WEIGHT GAIN

The oral contraceptive pill makes you retain water and also makes it easier for your body to convert food into fat. This means that if you are now maintaining your weight when eating 2000 calories/day and you start taking the Pill, you will have to reduce your intake by 10% or 200 calories/day. There are other side-effects of the Pill, too. If you feel any difference, tell your doctor. Since the Pill also affects your ability to absorb some nutrients, it would be wise to take a multiple vitamin/mineral tablet.

*I*NABILITY TO HANDLE CARBOHYDRATES

Everyone would like to find a medical reason for being overweight. When you go to the doctor for a checkup, you pray that she or he will discover some problem that can be fixed by taking a magic pill. Rarely do the tests find medical reasons for being overweight. (I know there are clinics that supply medications for weight loss, and I would like to warn you against them. The drugs prescribed have only temporary results and the people who take them do not lose weight any faster than others who do not. Unless there is a change in diet and lifestyle, no pill will have permanent results.)

There is a metabolic irregularity that has been found in some obese teenagers and adult women that causes them to store fat easily. Some females cannot process too many carbohydrates (bread, rice, beans, and pasta) at one time. While eating too much of any food causes weight gain, certain women cannot handle large amounts of starchy foods. Whether this condition causes obesity or obesity causes an intolerance to carbohydrates isn't clear. But if you feel you don't each that much, this may be one reason you are not losing weight. Are you eating all your food at once? Try eating smaller meals, limit your starches to one per meal, and resist that second helping.

*T*RADITION

This may or may not be a problem for you, at least not yet. In our society, women are usually in charge of buying, preparing, and cooking the food. Being around food for a good part of the day and having to think continually about it is a real disadvantage to anyone who is susceptible to gaining weight. If you already find yourself in the kitchen baking cakes and trying out recipes on your family, be aware that tastes and nibbles have calories too and they quickly add up.

3
Eating Disorders

Dieting has been taken to extremes by a large number of teenage girls. Only recently have we found out how many. Magazine articles written by celebrities like Jane Fonda point out the extent and seriousness of the disease. Few stories illustrate the potential dangers as clearly as the shocking story of Karen Carpenter's death several years ago. Carpenter, a famous singer, was a secret anorexic who died in her thirties from heart failure caused by years of starving herself. There are many books out now by professionals who understand what causes eating disorders. There are also accounts by girls who have personally struggled with them. If you think you might have a problem, get help as soon as possible. Don't wait.

Anorexia

The name *anorexia nervosa* means "nervous loss of appetite". The term is misleading because it is not the loss of appetite that forces girls to starve themselves. Rather, it is a voluntary decision not to eat. Strange as it sounds, food is not the anorexic's major problem. The individual has an unresolved emotional problem that needs professional help.

Anorexia is an eating disorder that seems to afflict a definite type of person. If you picture the perfect child, you will see a potential anorexic—obedient, cooperative, outgoing, bright, and eager to please. She is the top stream student, teacher's pet, and parent's delight. At least this is the person we see on the outside. On the inside, she is very different. She is not self-assured at all. She feels she is never good enough to meet either her parents' or her own standards, yet she doesn't know how to stop trying. She rebels by refusing to eat. This is the way she regains control—control over her life and over what is expected of her.

Anorexia is 10 to 20 times more common among women than men. Young women between the ages of 13 and 25 are most susceptible since they are at the age when they are struggling for independence from their parents. Many anorexics come from upper middle-class families and have parents who are over-protective, overly concerned, and overly ambitious for their child. While this scenario is common, other girls not in this category can also become anorexic.

Reasoning with an anorexic is next to impossible. You can tell her that she is too thin and her bones are sticking out, but she cannot see it. When she looks in a mirror, she doesn't see a gaunt, dangerously thin skeleton. She sees fat covering corners and crevices of her body that don't even exist. There is no sense of reality for this person. If anything, she is proud of her thinness because she thinks being trim is something that everybody else wants but only she can achieve.

Another paradox the anorexic exhibits is an obsession with food. While refusing all but bits and pieces, she also may be a gourmet cook who prepares delicious recipes for family and friends. She enjoys poring over cookbooks, clipping recipes, and making lists of every bit of food she eats with its caloric content. Despite her own malnutrition, she is often well-informed on nutritional matters.

The disorder is also characterized by relentless hyperactivity. In spite of the weakness associated with being severely underweight, the anorexic drives herself to unbelievable feats, to demonstrate that she has concontrol over her body. An anorexic girl may run 20 min a day, swim for one hour, and still be on time for morning aerobics. Her athletic endeavours, however, rarely include friends. Like eating, exercise is private and serious, not meant for fun and enjoyment.

Rarely do you see the anorexic sit back and relax. She is continually moving her body as if it were a crime to be still. I have watched two different anorexic girls in aerobics class. They would never "wind down" after working out. When the rest of us were stretching our tired muscles, they would still be bouncing at high intensity. Even in the sauna, they moved nervously around the room.

Are you or could you become anorexic?

- ▼ Are you a perfectionist? Do you need to be the best at everything you do?

- ▼ Do you set such high standards for yourself that they are almost impossible to attain?

- ▼ Do you go out of your way to please others?

- ▼ Have people told you that you are too thin?

- ▼ Are your parents over-protective or overly ambitious for you?

- ▼ Do you constantly think of food? Are you afraid of food?

- ▼ Do you eat less than 500 calories a day?

- ▼ Do you take diuretics or laxatives several times a week?

▼ Do you exercise for more than 2 hours a day, 6 days a week?

▼ Are your periods irregular or nonexistent?

▼ Do you have a hard time sitting down, reading, watching a film, or relaxing?

▼ Do you play games with your food? Count bites? Shove it around your plate rather than eat it?

▼ Have you given up seeing your friends?

Extreme weight loss is a serious medical problem. It results in malnutrition and all sorts of physical symptoms: interruption of menstrual periods, dry skin, skin discoloration, brittle nails and hair, loss of hair from the scalp, growth of long, fine hairs over the body, fluid retention, constipation, digestive problems, and anaemia. Eventually, the entire metabolic process slows down in an attempt to protect the individual from death. Blood pressure, pulse, and body temperature drop below normal.

Self-starvation is dangerous and deadly. If someone has mentioned to you that you have this problem and you don't believe them, look carefully at the list on pages 23–24 and see if any of the points apply to you.

If you recognize any of these traits, please talk to someone about it. You need professional help. Appendix B gives the phone number of the Eating Disorders Association. Call it now. Your health and happiness are important.

Nutritionally, I do have a few recommendations that will enable you to rebuild your health, yet not cause you to gain weight too fast.

Nutritional suggestions for anorexics

▼ Introduce foods in small amounts. If you are only eating once a day, try twice a day for a week, then three times a day for another week. It is better to eat several small meals throughout the day than three large meals.

▼ Choose high quality, low-fat foods; fresh fruit and vegetables, whole grain breads, cereals and pasta, and lean meats like chicken and fish.

▼ Drink diluted vegetable and fruit juices, mineral water, herb teas, and non- or low-fat milk.

▼ Have 1–2 tablespoons of vegetable oil each day. You can make it into a salad dressing.

▼ Take a multiple vitamin/mineral tablet each day.

▼ Take extra zinc (15 mg) twice a day.

BULIMIA

Like the anorexic, the bulimic individual tends to be achievement-oriented. She too is preoccupied with food and may have a fair understanding of nutrition. There is one major difference between the two: the anorexic is obsessed with getting thinner, and the bulimic is obsessed with avoiding weight gain. This may not seem like much of a difference, but it is. The anorexic won't eat because she feels any food will make her fat. The bulimic, on the other hand, is a compulsive eater, one who binges and then throws up so she won't gain weight. The bulimic is not excessively overweight, but she continually struggles with weight gain and is willing to do almost anything to avoid an extra pound. A bulimic may or may not become anorexic.

This strange word *bulimia* literally means "hunger like an ox". It describes people who "binge"—they uncontrollably eat an enormous amount of food at one time. They may sit down for a full meal and then follow it with three puddings, two bags of crisps, a dozen doughnuts, and a large pizza. The sheer amount of food intake, coupled with extreme guilt, then leads them to "purge": to get rid of all the food using laxatives, diuretics, or self-induced vomiting.

Expelling food unnaturally from the body on a regular basis is not only unhealthy, it can be extremely dangerous. Throwing up food does not allow for digestion or absorption of nutrients, so bulimics suffer from dietary deficiencies and imbalances. Over a period of time, forced elimination can result in the loss of important minerals, dehydration, chronic indigestion, permanently damaged teeth, swollen and infected salivary glands, a bleeding throat, premenstrual syndrome, and, in extreme cases, a ruptured oesophagus or stomach, and heart and kidney failure.

Bulimics often rely on laxatives and diuretics. Continued abuse of these medications causes additional problems and symptoms: abdominal pain, constipation, fatigue, headache, heart palpitations, kidney dysfunction, and muscle weakness.

Bulimia occurs most often in women who are:

▼ in their late teens or early 20s

▼ near normal in weight

▼ perfectionists

▼ emotionally insecure

▼ lacking in confidence

▼ continually afraid of getting fat

▼ constantly dieting

For most bulimics, however, the health problems are initially not as devastating as the mental anguish they experience after gorging and throwing up. They find it far easier to endure physical symptoms than to think someone may discover their horrible secret. The secretive nature of this problem makes diagnosis and therefore treatment difficult.

Again, I emphasize, if you know you have this problem, get professional help. Don't be ashamed—look in Appendix B for resources that can help you and call. You are worth it!

Compulsive eating

Compulsive overeaters, like bulimics, binge continuously. Unlike bulimics, however, they do not get rid of the food immediately by throwing up. They purge emotionally, punishing themselves for being a failure in this area.

It is normal to pig out at times. Many of us gorge at Christmas, and family parties, or when there is nothing better to do. This doesn't mean we are all unstable, abnormal, or bad. The difference between those of us who overeat occasionally and those who do it several times a week is that we in the first group don't take it personally. We brush it off. We may feel stuffed, but so what? It was no big deal and tomorrow we'll eat less. Perpetual overeaters see the binge as a personality flaw. They feel they are "bad" because they can't control their eating.

Some psychologists think people who overeat are really trying to do something good for themselves. They have problems they don't know how to deal with, so they use food to help them forget and to make them feel better. If this is true, the overeater needs to find out what is really bugging him or her. I suggest talking to your best friend, mum, sister, school counsellor, or adult friend to see if they can shed some light on how you might deal with your problem.

Maybe you have not made a connection between overeating and the way you feel. If not, I have an experiment for you. Write down how you feel before, during, and after you overeat. I know this seems like work, but it might help you figure out WHY you are overeating. Do you feel bored, angry, overtired, lonely, or what? I am not suggesting that you will stop overeating next week because you discovered, after you finished the last of the cake, that you were bored out of your skull or mad at your mum. But understanding why you binge is a start.

Another thing I want you to think about is being kinder to yourself when you *do* overeat. Forgive yourself. Know that you are working on your problem, but it will take time. As you realize what you are doing and why, you will get better at controlling yourself. You are not a bad person. In fact, you might be surprised to know how many other people do this too. Remember, if you are hiding this from your friends, don't you think some of them could be doing the same?

If the problem is just beginning, your chances of stopping it yourself are better. The following suggestions helped many compulsive eaters to control the bingeing attack. If even one suggestion works, you're a step closer to conquering the problem. Don't try to change more than one habit at a time. And, always start with the easiest first. When you feel successful with one area, try another suggestion.

Suggestions for compulsive overeaters

1. Begin by **observing your eating habits**. Write down what, when, and how you feel when you overeat. Do this for several weeks, so you can see if you always overeat for the same or for different reasons. There may be more than one trigger for bingeing. Do you overeat every day or only when you are upset? Do you raid the fridge at night, or in the afternoon, or when the "soaps" are on—when?

2. Once you have identified patterns, **make a list of things you could do during those moments you are most susceptible.** Maybe you could walk the dog, call a friend, go to a film, rent a video, read a magazine or book, go shopping, or whatever you like to do most. Try to rearrange your schedule so that you will not be faced with the temptation.

3. **Plan one day's eating at a time.** What are you going to do tomorrow? When will you be eating? What are you most likely to eat? Is tomorrow going to be a fun day or might it be one of those days when you are going to be tempted to binge? What else could you do to make it a more fun day? At the end of the day, look at your plan. Did you do what you thought you were going to do? Were there surprises? If you did overeat, what could you have done differently? Don't feel bad if you didn't follow your plan. Remember, you're just starting this and it takes time to change old habits.

4. **There are no forbidden foods.** If you eat a small amount of the food you really want when you want it, you are less likely to overeat something else. If you crave a Mars bar but get yogurt because that is better for you and has fewer calories, you may just

end up eating both anyway. Sounds familiar?

5. When you want to cut down on calories to lose weight, **use the "better than" approach**. Even though I believe there is no such thing as "bad" food, try to learn to enjoy foods that are lower in calories and more nutritious. When you are hungry and not craving anything in particular, a piece of fruit is better than a cake. Or a cereal bar is better than a Mars bar. Sometimes this works, and sometimes nothing will replace that Mars bar. Use this approach when you can, and you may be surprised that you will start doing it more and more.

6. **Eat with friends.** Many people who are overweight, or think they are, do not eat in public. Then when they get home, they eat anything that's not nailed down. It could be two to three times what they would have eaten if they had eaten with their friends. Because they feel fat, some people want to show the world they are trying to cut back. Besides, they feel they don't deserve to enjoy food if they are fat. Denying yourself fun and the social enjoyment of eating leads to solitary overeating and self-hatred. Go ahead and have fun in public.

7. **Pay attention when you eat.** Eat when you are sitting down at the table. Foods eaten standing up or in a car don't count, do they? There are no calories in a biscuit gobbled up as you are running out of the door, right? Wrong. When you eat, be serious and sit down. Look at the food. Are you hungry? Do you really want it? Know *that* you are eating and *what* you are eating. Is it good? If not, don't waste your calories.

8. **Don't eat if you are angry, upset, sad, or overly**

emotional. Wait until you can enjoy your food. Drink something like water or a diet drink instead.

9. **When you "blow it," and you will, you blow it only for that moment.** One slip doesn't mean you have to give up on the whole day. Get right back on course. And, whatever you do, don't punish yourself for your choice. Use it as a learning experience. Why did it happen and what can you do next time? Rather than give yourself a guilt trip, plan what you will do next time. Allow yourself to fail.

10. **Be aware of when you are really hungry.** What does it feel like? You want to eat when you feel true hunger. Don't you enjoy food more when you are famished? If you're not all that hungry, do something to take your mind off food. If you are ready to eat, look at your food, smell it, touch it, taste it. Eat slowly and love each bite. Turn off the TV when you're eating so you can really concentrate on the experience of chewing and swallowing.

Winning the battle of overeating is not easy, but it is possible. It begins with an awareness of the situation, admitting you have the problem, and developing your own plan to change it. Once you do this, you are already on your way to self-control. You will not conquer it overnight, so don't get discouraged and think it is hopeless. Expect small, short victories. Each time you overcome one potential binge, you are one step closer to being in charge of your life. Congratulate yourself!

4
How *Not* to Diet

Strange as it may sound, many teenagers don't have a real weight problem until they start to diet. Who do you know who isn't following some weird new system? Fad diets are not new. In my lifetime I have seen the grapefruit and vinegar diet, the egg diet, the banana diet, the rice diet, and the high protein diet. It doesn't take a medical mind to think up a fad. Just come up with something unusual and you too can be the next weight-loss guru.

All you probably want to know is, will the diet work? The answer is, yes, probably. Whenever you lower your calories beyond a certain point, you are going to lose weight. So what's the problem, if it works? Think about it. How many times have you or your mum tried something like this? I mention your mum because she and her friends have probably experimented with more diets than you and your friends. Ask them how many times they have lost and regained the same amount of weight. A few? Several? So why are they going through this torture again? Because the fat didn't stay off. They followed a temporary diet and got temporary results.

I am constantly amazed that people go back to the same diet after they have regained their weight. Learn from the others who have tried and failed and don't waste your money. I've said it before and I'll say it again. Most commercial programmes and fad diets are not successful at keeping the weight off. The only method that really works is a change in lifestyle habits.

Semi-starvation fad diets, commercial diets, protein drinks, diet pills, and vitamins are commonly used today to speed up weight loss. Each comes with its own set of problems. Be suspicious of the so-called fast weight-loss advertisements. Remember, the faster it comes off, the faster it will probably come back on. "Yo-yo" dieting is not fun and it may harm you both physically and emotionally.

Very low calorie fad diets

The fad diets that we have all tried at one time or another are usually a form of semi-starvation. Whether you are drinking a chalky liquid or limiting your meals to lettuce leaves and diet drinks, most likely you are drastically restricting your calories. The body interprets this lack of food as starvation. While you think you're losing weight quickly, what you're really doing is setting up a condition in your body which will actually cause you to make fat more easily.

When you severely deprive your body of calories, the organs and glands slow down so you can conserve all of your energy just to stay alive. Muscle tissue is burned, while the fat hangs on tightly as your last energy reserve. You may be eating less food, but you are not burning it very efficiently, and when you do eat, your body just wants to store the calories because it doesn't know when the next meal is coming. The result is a lowered metabolic rate. As soon as you start eating hamburgers and fries again, those familiar pounds find their way back—faster than before.

With self-starvation also comes a loss of appetite. You can train yourself so well to eat according to a specific schedule that you lose your natural internal cues for hunger and fullness. Some people I know have had a very difficult time relearning how to enjoy food after going on a strict diet.

Another precaution: very low calorie diets often lead to bingeing. There is much evidence that starving yourself and even going all day without eating may cause overeating. We think our frequent trips to the biscuit tin come from lack of self-control when, in fact, they may be the body telling us we're not feeding it properly.

Over time, extremely low-calorie diets may cause physical symptoms like fatigue, sleep disturbances, dry skin and hair, constipation, cold sensitivity, and depression. Never trust a diet that goes below 1000 calories per day. For teenagers, a safer weight-loss programme should be around 1200 to 1500 calories per day.

Skipping Meals

Many teenagers and adults will go all day without eating as a means of controlling their weight. They avoid breakfast and lunch and then make up for it at suppertime. They rationalize eating so much because they feel they deserve it—they fasted all day. But even if you only eat 1000 calories a day, getting them all in one meal causes weight gain, not weight loss. This really has been proven. So, once again, this is not an effective way to lose weight.

Studies have shown that you can lose weight faster and can take in more calories by eating several small meals throughout the day. Skipping meals has the same effect as starving the body. It slows the metabolism 3% to 4% and can make you feel sluggish. Did you know that you actually burn calories digesting and absorbing food? I know how busy you are and how frantic your mornings can get, but if you seriously want to lose some weight, grab an apple, a banana, or a piece of whole wheat toast before leaving the house.

COMMERCIAL PROGRAMMES

Don't waste your parents' money—or your own—on commercial diets. I have worked for some of the top diets advertised on TV, and I have seen first-hand the number of people who returned because they gained all their weight back. For the most part, these diets encourage your dependence on their food. Most important, they don't teach you how to live in the real world of parties, restaurants, and holidays.

LIQUID DIETS

I don't believe that liquid diets are the answer either, again because of my experience working for one of the top programmes. I saw people lose, gain, lose, gain, lose, and gain. The prize dieters who lost the fastest also gained back their weight the fastest. I always marvelled that the "cheaters" were the ones who maintained their weight the longest because they were already creating new ways of eating. The others only knew how to be "on" a diet or "off" a diet. There was no middle ground.

Liquid diets are a very restrictive and extreme way to lose weight, especially for a teenager. To sip on a diet drink while others are munching on fries takes a special type of individual. Even the most "mature" of my teenagers were not successful doing the drink thing. Even though many of the canned meal replacements are quite tasty, going without solids is boring and can be harmful. I've seen many people who lose their appetite for food and find it hard going back to the real thing.

On the positive side, diet drinks are generally low in calories and fat and they're very convenient. If they are used to replace one meal or a snack, they can be integrated into your diet. It is certainly better to have a nutritional drink than to go without eating at all. Diet drinks can be good substitutes for high fat snacks and treats. My main concern is that you eat at least two solid meals a day.

*P*ILLS AND DIET AIDS

Pills, potions, and diet aids to speed up the weight-loss process have been around forever. And do they ever sell! I guess we're all gullible when it comes to the quick and easy methods. But the hard truth is: there are no magic pills to make dieting easy. In fact, anything that promises to take more than two pounds off in one week should be avoided like the plague. Don't waste your money trying these schemes, no matter which Hollywood star endorses them.

Uppers

Most of the diet pills you get from the doctor or borrow from your friends are drugs known as amphetamines or "uppers". These pills were originally prescribed for depressed patients, to raise their spirits. They make you feel unusually alert and energetic. At the same time, your appetite goes away. Maybe this sounds pretty good to you, but there is a dark side. In order to stay "high", you need to keep taking the pills or the effects wear off. When they do, you go from feeling "up" to feeling down, sad, and nervous. The only way to feel good again is to take more pills. Get the picture? You're ADDICTED. The potential for abuse with diet pills is very strong, so, if you're smart, you won't start.

Appetite suppressants

You can go into any chemist or supermarket and find an entire shelf filled with over-the-counter diet pills. Some of the appetite suppressants are chemically related to "uppers" and have similar reactions; however, they generally are not as strong and don't have such dramatic side-effects. They may still cause reactions like insomnia, restlessness, nausea, nervousness, and headache.

Some appetite suppressants are decongestants, much like cold and allergy remedies. They also may be combined with caffeine (for pep) and a local anaesthetic (to dull the taste buds). None are completely safe or free from side-effects. Just because you can buy them yourself, don't think they are harmless.

Diuretics or water pills

Water pills are taken to get rid of extra water in your body. Some people take them because it appears they have lost weight when they step on the scales. Some women often take them the week before their periods to relieve bloating. Don't be fooled by these pills. The scales may show a few pounds lighter, but as soon as you drink a glass of liquid, the pounds come right back. Water pills also increase premenstrual syndrome symptoms. If your body tends to hold water (you can tell this if your rings and shoes feel tight), watch your salt and sugar intake and drink plenty of water. I know it sounds strange, but drinking more water helps to relieve the puffiness.

Other diet aids

Diet aids include wafers, sweets, and nutrients that you eat between meals or an hour before you eat a meal so you will not be as hungry. Do they cut down your appetite? Yes. But so will an apple, an orange, yogurt, or a cracker—and they're much cheaper. Recently, health advocates have joined the diet bandwagon and found so-called natural remedies that depress the appetite or prevent food from being digested. I'm referring to the starch blockers, grapefruit pills, amino acids, and fibre tablets. If you had to choose between these and the medications, I would say the nutrients are safer for most people. But again, why not eat the grapefruit or some natural fibre rather than relying on pills? Food tastes better and really is natural.

By the way, don't be misled by the label "natural". It doesn't mean very much these days. In fact, it doesn't always mean that the food is healthy, without additives, or low in calories. Vitamins and minerals too, must be taken with caution. In large amounts they can act like a drug and may cause harmful reactions.

Pills and diet aids are not the way to permanent weight loss. They may provide a small benefit, but the potential for harm is too great for them to be a realistic alternative. And, of course, they don't teach you how to keep your weight off.

5

Dieting Starts in the Mind, Not the Mouth

You are now ready to start. You've psyched yourself up to do whatever it takes to get this weight off. This is good, because dieting really does start in the mind and not in the mouth. You need to want to lose weight badly enough to change some of your habits. Notice I said SOME, not all. You don't have to give up totally everything you enjoy. But obviously, some things have to be changed.

Changing habits involves thought and planning. That is why you need to examine what you are doing right now so you can make the changes that will be necessary to reach your goal. You may think this is dumb and a waste of time, but it's not. Before you go on a trip you need to plan your route. I can help you by mapping out different ways to go. You pick the specific course.

I am going to take you through a series of steps to get you thinking about your eating patterns. Once you see exactly what you are doing, the plan will be clearer.

I want you to consider several things about yourself and then write out your responses. Putting your thoughts down on paper makes them more real.

Most of all, be HONEST with your answers. No one will see them. You won't be graded. This is all meant to help you understand *who* you are and *what* you want.

How do you feel about being overweight?

We can only make changes when we are really ready. If your weight is not a problem for you and you're not unhappy about it, wait until you are. Maybe your mother nags you about it, your little sister teases you, and the relatives make well-meaning comments. You think you should do something, but for some reason you're just not motivated. Then wait. Don't lose weight for anyone but yourself. When the decision is yours, the process will come easier. In fact, if you are not ready for the commitment, it just won't work.

How do you feel about your weight? Even if you think it is not worth dwelling on, do this exercise. Be honest. You may find out something about yourself. I'll start you out with comments I've heard from other teenagers, then you fill in your own thoughts. I've heard many teenagers say: I feel

- ▼ ugly: I can't wear the latest styles, and the clothes I do wear look sloppy

- ▼ self-conscious: I don't fit in with the other kids

- ▼ embarrassed: I hate going to parties or going shopping with friends because they all look better than me

- ▼ angry: my mother tells me not to eat fattening things and then she brings them home

- ▼ envious: my best friend is a stick

- ▼ frustrated: I want to lose weight, but I want to eat with my friends and have fun too

▼ insecure: people talk about me and think I'm fat

▼ bad: the boys don't ask me out

How I feel about my weight now

1. _____

2. _____

3. _____

4. _____

5. _____

If you could close your eyes and magically lose that layer of fat, how would you feel? How would your life change? What would you wear? What would you be doing with your friends? Where might you go? How would life be different? Close your eyes and picture yourself the way you want to look. Is it hard? Keep trying. Glance at the following list if you want some ideas, then write down the way you see your ideal self.

If I were at my goal weight, I would be:

▼ looking good

▼ feeling good about myself

▼ confident

▼ popular

▼ going out all the time

▼ wearing fabulous clothes

▼ dating every night

▼ showing off my body, not covering it up

▼ friendlier

Now it's your turn.

If I were at my goal weight, I would be:

1. _____
_____
2. _____
_____
3. _____
_____
4. _____
_____
5. _____
_____

Have you ever thought that the reason you haven't lost weight is that you might be afraid of changing your personality, or that you might have to make new decisions about your social life and how people respond to you? Maybe you think that if you were thinner, you might be:

▼ too different (I know who I am now)

▼ noticed (how would I handle that?)

▼ friendless (my friends say they like me as I am)

▼ sexy (I wouldn't know how to act)

▼ responsible (I would have to do those things I said I would do when I lost weight)

▼ like everyone else (I like being different)

Maybe you are not ready to make these changes yet. This might really be scary for you. Could you talk to someone about it? Do it now.

Feeling good about yourself

Scientific studies have shown that people are more likely to take weight off and keep it off when they feel good about themselves. I know this is easier said than done. Even before you plan your food or exercise programme, I want you to think about and write down your best qualities (hair, eyes, legs, smile, personality). Sometimes it's hard to come up with a best quality, so ask a friend. Maybe your good points include things you cannot see: kindness, generosity, friendliness, artistic or musical skills, being smart or funny. Write down everything you like about yourself.

The best things about me are:

1. _____
_____

2. _____

3. _____

4. _____

5. _____

Was this section difficult for you? Maybe you don't feel all that great about the way you look and who you are. Let's do something about that right now, today. What would make you feel better about your image? What can you do to improve ONE thing that really bugs you?

Need suggestions? How about updating your wardrobe? So you don't look good in tank tops and shorts. Then don't buy them. There are fashionable styles for all sizes and shapes. I know you would rather wait until you have lost some weight and then buy new clothes, but this may be an excuse to postpone becoming the person you want to be. If you feel better about the way you look *now*, you are more likely to move more quickly towards your goal. When you look and feel good, it becomes infectious and you want more of it.

Change should be gradual, so let's start right now with the small stuff. Small successes lead to bigger successes.

What changes could you make at this time? How about a new hairstyle, acrylic fingernails, or new make-up? And don't forget to look at your posture. At the risk of sounding like a parent, do you stand tall with your head up and your shoulders back? Or are you slumped over and always looking at your feet? Practise walking upright. Look as if you have somewhere important to go (even if you don't). This alone will keep people wondering what you have done to yourself, when you haven't spent a penny. As my good friend Bobbe Sommer says, "Fake it till you make it."

Don't just concentrate on cosmetic changes. What can you do to be a better person on the INSIDE? Have you ever thought of joining a group or volunteering for an organization? There are so many people in need. And there is nothing that makes a person feel better than helping others. School clubs, church groups, and other youth groups are good places to start.

What about learning a new hobby, sport, or activity? What are your interests? Try something new. Once you add more variety to your life, eating will not have the importance it has now. If you are serious about losing weight, begin by making yourself feel better in other areas of your life.

*W*HY I WANT TO LOSE WEIGHT

Why do you want to lose weight? Do you think this is a stupid question, or do you think the reasons are too obvious to warrant an answer? If you have been on any diet, you know the first few days are the easiest because you are strongly motivated. You have no desire to munch and you are a tower of strength when it comes to turning down fries. A few days later the story changes. You're sick of cottage cheese and protein drinks, you're craving a quarter-pounder, and you have no idea why you ever wanted to diet at all. During these "down" moments, a reminder like the one you are going to make will be helpful. If you can refresh your memory with all the reasons why you want to change your habits, your chances of giving in to temptation are greatly reduced.

It is much easier to control what you eat when you are concentrating on why you want to lose weight. When you can actually picture in your mind the results of your efforts, you are more likely to stay on course. On the other hand, it is next to impossible to resist an ice-cream cone when you are imagining how good it might taste. With this in mind I want you to put down on paper all the reasons that you can think of why you want this weight off. If you can think of more later, add them. To get you started, here are some reasons to lose weight that teenagers have told me:

- ▼ I want to look better

- ▼ I don't want to feel uncomfortable around my friends

- ▼ I want to wear lycra

- ▼ I want to sit on my boyfriend's lap and not feel heavy

- ▼ I want to walk past a window and like the reflection

- ▼ I want my mum and dad to be proud of me

- ▼ I want to feel good about myself.

Why I really want to lose weight

1. _____

2. _____

3. _____

4. _____

5. _____

6._____

7._____

8._____

Design your dreams

There are mental exercises or tricks you can use that will help make dieting or changing your habits easier. You have just completed one. You thought about and wrote down why it is important for you to lose weight. Take a look at that list again. Read it, and then imagine yourself as the person you described. Now go over the list you filled out a few pages ago, the one that states how you would feel at your goal weight. Close your eyes and see that person. Really get into it and *feel* how you want to look. Do you have a clear picture in your mind? Is it hard to imagine? Does your mind keep telling you that you can never look like that? Keep trying. It will get easier. To help you out, do the following exercises. You will need to use the lists you created, so if you have not completed them, go back and do them now.

Mental imagining

It is easier and faster to achieve a goal if you can picture it in your mind. So, I want you to do what you just did in the preceding paragraph, only this time concentrate for more than a few seconds on your "image". Sit down in a comfortable position and shut your eyes. Breathe in and out deeply 10 times, counting to five slowly with each breath. Feel your whole body relax. Start with your toes. Move up to your feet, ankles, calves, thighs, bottom, back, stomach, chest, shoulders, arms, neck, and head. Relax each and every part of your body. Now that you are totally quiet, I want you to think about your goals and the way you want to look and feel. Get specific. What are you wearing? Who are you with? What are you doing? How do you walk, talk, carry yourself? See yourself the way you want to be, and in time you will be the way you see yourself. Continue breathing in and out deeply another 10 times. Open your eyes and know that your goal is beginning to happen. Do this once a day until your goal is reached.

Thought for the day

Another technique uses the same lists. This time write one goal—one reason why you want to lose weight—on a small index card. Reword it so it reads like a positive thought for the day. Take the card with you for a week and read it at least five times during the day. This is another way to keep you focused on your goal. At the end of the week, make up a new card with another goal and do the same the following week. Continue until all of your goals are used up and then start all over again or make up some new ones. If you have trouble coming up with positive thoughts, here are some suggestions.

- ▼ I am in control of my life

- ▼ I feel great about myself

- ▼ I like who I am

- ▼ I look good

- ▼ I have a lot of energy

▼ I am confident

▼ I am healthy

▼ I am getting better and better each day

▼ I am in control of my eating

▼ I am active and I like to be out doing things

Goal board

There is one more exercise that I find very useful to help me see myself the way I want to be. It's called a goal board, and on it I put everything I like to do, want to be, or hope to become. By keeping that mental image in my mind, I find I am more likely to make the choices I need to achieve my goals.

To make the board you need a few items: a piece of poster board (mine is 60 cm x 100 cm), scissors, a stick of glue and several magazines. Flip through the magazines and find words, phrases, or pictures that express you, your ambitions, your dreams and wishes. Cut them out and paste them on your goal board in any fashion you want. There is no right or wrong way to do it.

Should I tell you what mine looks like? In the centre I have pictures of my family and words like "together", "love", "secure", and "support". In one corner I have health goals: pictures of carrots, a green salad, and fresh fruits. I have several exercise-type pictures—women jogging and doing aerobics. The words I found for this section include: "love your body", "fit and trim", "calories", and "energy blast your day". I also have career goals, wishes, and wants. I have scenes of London and other places, aeroplanes, and beautiful hotels. Expressing my goals are phrases like "brilliant achievement", "enjoy life", "quality work", "experience God's love", and "always improve". Get the idea?

Looking at this board every day reminds you of your goals and keeps you focused. Be creative. Add to it as you find pictures that better represent you and what you want. Remember, concentrating on your goals will help you to achieve them.

6
Exercise and Physical Activity

Do you want a sure way to lose weight—one that doesn't require super will-power or lunches of apples and Diet Coke? One that is fun, gives you energy, makes you feel better, and builds your self-confidence? One that keeps your weight down forever and allows you to eat more of the food you like?

There is such a magic formula, and it's called EXERCISE.

Researchers have found that more people are overweight because of inactivity than overeating. Do you get a lift to school or to the shops rather than walking? Do you take escalators instead of stairs? Do you pay your brother to do your chores? If you just made some of these small changes in your daily activity level, you could lose up to a pound a week! Then you wouldn't have to worry so much about what you eat.

Most people start to diet by cutting down on the calories they take in. But losing weight would be much better—and much easier—if they just increased their activity level. If you had to choose diet or exercise as a weight control method, I would say go for the exercise. I'm not suggesting that you forget about what you eat. But I do want you to see the terrific value of increased physical activity and regular exercise.

Why exercise?

What is so great about exercise anyway? I don't want to bore you with all the physiological changes that occur in the body when you exercise, but knowing something about the very practical benefits of exercise may convince you that it's well worth the time and effort.

Exercise burns calories

The best reason to exercise is to burn off calories. When you sit and watch TV or talk on the phone, you are burning about 120 calories per hour. This isn't much when you consider one scoop of Haagen-Dazs has double that. Just casually walking along the street burns 240 calories per hour, so even this minimal activity is an improvement over lounging about. Now, if you really get ambitious and decide to clean your room, wash the car, or vacuum the house, you could polish off 300 calories (enough to cover the leftover cake). Increasing your activity level by walking more, taking the stairs instead of the escalator, or moving more in general could mean a loss of an extra pound a week, 4 pounds a month, and a grand total of 48 pounds a year!

You can really see a difference in your body when you start an aerobic activity like fast walking, bike riding, or aerobic dancing. These burn 400–500 calories per hour. If you start something you like that uses up this many calories, you may never have to worry about food again.

Exercise burns fat

Exercise produces enzymes that help your body burn fat. Overweight people have hormones and enzymes that store fat easily and efficiently. Aerobic exercise is the best way to change the metabolism from fat-STORING to fat-BURNING. Pills and diet aids do not burn fat. Exercise does.

Exercise speeds up metabolism

Exercise speeds up your metabolic rate so you burn calories faster even when your body is at rest. Cutting calories way down does the reverse and lowers your metabolic rate.

Exercise builds muscles

Continuous exercise builds up your muscles. Muscle burns calories; fat just sits there. The more muscles you have, the more calories you are going to burn. This is why most blokes can eat two full meals and still not gain weight. It's also why they can lose it more easily than girls, who naturally store fat in their bodies. Building your muscles also will enable you to eat more. Fortunately, it is not unfeminine for women to develop their muscles, and we can change our bodies from fat-storing to fat-burning by building up our muscle mass.

Exercise controls appetite

Most people notice that they are not hungry after exercising regularly. That's because fat is released into the bloodstream as sugar, so you feel full. Also, after regular exercise, the appetite regulator in your brain resets itself, so your body becomes more tuned in to your hunger needs. In other words, you will be more conscious of your real feelings of hunger as opposed to the false hunger signals. Let me warn you that this process takes time to work, so when you first start exercising you may experience increased hunger after exercise. Soon, however, exercise will decrease your urge to eat.

Exercise reduces calories absorbed

Food passes through the digestive system faster when you are active than it does when you are inactive. As a result, a smaller percentage of your daily calories is stored as fat. For example, the average person processes a meal in about 24 hours. In obese people, it may take twice as long to digest, meaning that there is more time for the calories to be stored as fat. Well-trained athletes only keep food in their system for 4 to 6 hours. It literally doesn't have a chance to stick to their thighs!

Exercise helps to feel good

Exercise takes away anxiety and depression. Many illnesses are related to stress. If you feel tense and anxious, you will find that after exercising regularly you will feel calmer and more relaxed. Exercise has been used in clinics as a behaviour substitute for compulsive eating. If you are prone to bingeing, try working out more often.

Exercise fosters discipline and self-esteem

A number of positive psychological changes occur when you confront a challenge and overcome it. If you have been inactive, your challenge may be exercise. Sticking to a programme, whatever it is, will give you a sense of accomplishment and boost your self-image. When you feel better about yourself, you will find it easier to stay on course.

Aerobic Exercise

When I use the word exercise, sometimes I'm referring to physical activity and sometimes I'm talking about "aerobic" exercise. Don't get confused. Physical activity is basically being more active, like walking more. It's a good practice for all of us and does burn calories. Aerobic exercise is different. It is a specific type of exercise that burns fat most efficiently and makes weight loss quicker and easier.

"Aerobics" is a popular term, and you might associate it with an aerobics dance class or videotape. Those are aerobic workouts, but they are not the only way to achieve aerobic benefits. You can do many things: walk, jog, bike ride, swim, skip, or climb stairs. The most important thing you want to consider is, do you LIKE doing the activity enough that you will do it at least four times a week? You don't just have to choose one kind, either. Actually, it's better to do a variety of exercises so you work different muscles. The word aerobic simply means "oxygen in the air". As you exercise, your heart rate goes up, which brings more oxygen to your muscles so they can work. This type of exercise is the most efficient way to reduce fat in your body. If you overdo your workout, you force the muscles to work without oxygen (anaerobically), they will feel pain and your body will not get the same benefit as it did when you were exercising with air (aerobically).

To get all the aerobic benefits from your workout session, there are specific things you need to know. The activity you choose must be done non-stop for 20 to 30 minutes, at least four times a week, and within a specified range of intensity called your "training zone". If you leave out any part, you won't get the full benefit.

Let me repeat the criteria for an aerobic activity. It must be done:

▼ 20–30 minutes non-stop

▼ 4 times a week minimum

▼ within your training zone

What is this training zone? Very simply, it is the amount of effort you need to raise your heart rate to 140–160 beats per minute while doing the exercise. What this means is that when you are jogging, dancing, or walking, you want to make sure your heart is pumping hard enough to get up to this level, but not so hard that you go overboard. When you're exercising within this range, you're burning fat and not muscle, and your dieting efforts are much easier.

The first workout

Suppose that you are going to follow a programme of aerobic exercise. Let's start with Day One and I'll take you through your first session. Let's say you don't know what you want to try. I suggest fast walking. It's easy to do, and you don't have to buy anything for it. Just wear a decent pair of shoes with some arch support.

Before you leave the house, do two things. First, get a watch with a seconds hand so you can take your pulse about five minutes into the workout. Second, warm up your body by gently bending, twisting, and stretching for about 10 minutes. This is important, so don't leave it out.

Are you ready? Start walking slowly, gradually increasing your speed until you feel your heart is beating rapidly. Try talking. If no one is with you, talk out loud to yourself. If you feel too out of breath, slow down until you can carry on a conversation. And don't pay any attention to the people staring at you! Keep this pace for about five minutes.

As you continue to walk, take your pulse. You can find it on your wrist, about an inch from the base of your thumb, or on your neck, an inch below your ear. Remember what your pulse is supposed to be per minute? Right, between 140 and 160 beats. But that takes too long too count. So, let's make it easy. Take it for six seconds and add a nought. Your number now should be 14 to 16. Easier, isn't it? Is your number in this range? Is it higher? If it is, slow down for the end of your workout. Is it lower? Then pick up the pace.

You won't have to take your pulse every time you go out and you won't have to talk to yourself each time either. Once you've done it a few times, you will know what it feels like to be within your training range. Exercising at your training range for 20–30 minutes is ideal, but any amount of exercise counts. When you have finished your workout, slow down gradually and end by stretching, so your muscles won't be sore the next day.

If walking seems too boring, ask a friend to join you. Just remember, her or his pace and training rate may be different. Many people take their headphones along to relieve the boredom. Still not your thing? Would you feel better in a structured aerobics class? Or how about checking out some of the exercise videos, to see if they would work for you? How about bike riding, climbing stairs, or skipping with a rope. There are many options. Just make sure you like what you choose.

Why people stop

When people start a fitness programme—and I'm not just talking about teenagers—they do one of two things wrong. Either they go at it too vigorously and burn out, or they don't work hard enough and get discouraged because the results take too long.

It could be that this has already happened to you in

the past. You got excited at the prospect of losing weight. You begged your mum for the blank cheque to get the right clothes, shoes, and equipment. Day One you hurried off to the gym or hit the streets. In order to get this activity over as soon as possible, you ploughed into it full steam ahead. Three minutes later the steam evaporated, you were huffing and puffing and ready to call it quits. You rested for a minute, then ploughed into it again until exhaustion took over. Stop, start, stop, start. Your muscles ached, your joints cried out, and above all, you were NOT having fun.

Or maybe you gave in to a parent's or friend's nagging and half-heartedly strolled around the park once a week, or signed up for a class but couldn't seem to make it to all the sessions. You vowed that exercise was not your thing, never was, and never would be. Does this ring a bell? If it does, don't give up yet. Take a chance, and try again.

You must prepare your body to work out. Ease into it. Don't shock it. Get used to the way you feel when your pulse is increased. Does it seem uncomfortable? Maybe you should ease up. Feel your muscles. Are they tight? Consciously relax, and they will loosen up. Whether you are starting to change your eating habits or you are beginning to exercise, do it gradually and steadily. Your chances of staying with it improve. Do it right. Take it slowly. Stick with it. You and your body will be glad you did.

When you start your exercise programme, start slowly. Don't jump into one hour of rigorous sweating the first day. Get used to the idea, and if 10 minutes is all you can handle, fine. Build on that. It is better to adjust to the idea and new feelings and build on that gradually rather than burn yourself out after a few times. But do make a commitment, and even if you miss a few sessions, keep your promise to yourself. Sticking to your goal will make you feel better both physically AND emotionally.

How many calories am I burning?

The chart below lists both aerobic exercises and everyday physical activities, and shows how many calories you can burn off by doing them. You can figure out what you do or are going to do and how many calories you want to burn off. If you can't hack 30 minutes of exercise, don't despair. Start with 10 minutes, or even 5 if you want, and add some more daily activities. Just start.

Do you need to exercise to lose weight and keep it off? You'd better believe it. Exercise makes all the difference in the world.

Calories burned for 30 minutes of activity
Based on a person weighing 150 pounds. If you weigh more, you burn more calories; if you weigh less, you burn fewer calories.

Activity	*Calories for 30 minutes*
Aerobic classes	210
Badminton	200
Basketball	280
Canoeing (recreational)	90
Cleaning house (steady movement)	125
Climbing hills (steady pace)	250
Cycling (5.5 mph)	130
(9.5 mph)	200
(13 mph)	240
Football	270
Golf (walking)	180
Gymnastics	180
Horse riding (walking)	85
(cantering)	240
Judo/Karate	400
Piano playing	80
Rowing (machine)	210

Activity	*Calories for 30 minutes*
Running (11.5 min/mile)	280
(9.0 min/mile)	400
(6.0 min/mile)	520
Shopping	120
Skating (vigorously)	300
(moderately)	160
Skiing (cross-country)	300
(downhill)	200
Squash	440
Swimming (moderate)	280
Table tennis (recreational)	220
Tennis	240
Volleyball (moderate)	100
(vigorous)	280
Walking (3 mph)	130
(4 mph)	200
(stairs)	300
Weight training	240
Writing	60

7
Designing Your Own Diet

Finally, we've come to the DIET part! Don't panic. It's not going to be as bad as you imagine. You don't have to give up everything you like, you don't have to eat strange, tasteless foods, and you can still go out with your friends. Does it sound too good to be true? It's no trick. This diet is easy, it's realistic, and it works.

It works because you learn what you are doing now that keeps you from losing weight and what you need to do to start losing weight. More important, *you* decide how to make this happen. The only person controlling your diet is you.

A big difference between this programme and most others is that it's not meant to happen overnight. No matter what you hear or read, you can't burn fat while you sleep or in a few days. I know many programmes promise you quick weight loss. Don't be fooled. If you do lose weight rapidly, it is not fat weight and it won't stay off. On the other hand, if you lose one or even two pounds a week slowly, by changing some of your daily habits, your chances of keeping the pounds off are good.

Basically, the safe teenager diet centres around the calories you eat and the calories you burn off. Don't let the experts convince you that calories don't count. They do—especially fat calories. Yes, there are other factors involved in weight loss, but the bottom line is: CALORIES IN, CALORIES OUT.

It is my experience that most people are totally

unaware of the number of calories of fat they take in in one day. When people find out, it's almost always a shock. So start by figuring out what you eat and the number of calories in these foods, then you can decide how you want to lower that number. There are several ways:

1. You can replace the high-calorie foods with low-calorie foods

2. You can cut down on the amount of food (just eat less)

3. Do both of the above—or vary your plan by doing some of each.

*P*LAN OF ACTION

You may know exactly how much weight you want to lose, or you may have no idea at all. It doesn't really matter on this plan. You're on this programme to create habits that will keep your weight off for life, and as you get closer to your goal, you will know what feels and looks good. Don't get hung up on numbers. When you feel comfortable with the way you look, stop. But be careful to maintain the habits that got you to your goal.

Your weekly weight-loss goal should be no more than one or two pounds. Doesn't sound like much? If you were paying several hundred pounds to go to a commercial weight-loss programme, that is what they would expect too. Remember, that's 4 to 8 pounds a month or 8 to 16 pounds in two months and 48 pounds in six months. Sound any better?

The amount of food and the number of calories that you are able to eat on a diet depends upon your individual metabolism and activity level. Normally, female teenagers consume about 3,000 calories a day and males can often go above 5,000 a day without gaining weight. But, like I said, this can vary. To lose weight then, you need to go below this number. However, under no circumstances are you to eat less than 1,200–1,500 calories a day. Not only is this unhealthy and unsafe, you won't lose your fat any faster.

Plan 1

There are two ways to go about planning a diet. The first is to keep your calories under a certain number or within a specified range each day.

If you count calories, you would keep them between 1,200 and 1,500 per day. I don't expect you to know how many calories you are eating now, so one of your projects is to figure this out. It's not difficult. The tables in Appendix A will help you. Then you decide how you want to make the numbers work out.

Daily ranges of calories

Females	1200–1500
Males	1500–1800

Plan 2

The second way to design a diet plan is to find ways to cut out a certain number of calories from your present diet. A reasonable number would be between 500 and 1,000 calories per day. This may be easier than Plan 1, since you have fewer numbers to worry about. If you choose this way, you still need to know how many calories are in what you are now eating. Then you can go about looking for ways to cut down that number.

Before we continue, do you remember how many calories make up one pound of fat?

3500 CALORIES = 1 POUND OF FAT

You don't have to get hung up with the maths, but understand this so you know what you need to do to reach your goal. If you want to lose one pound of fat this week, you need to shave 3500 calories off your present diet for the week. This amounts to 500 calories a day. If you're looking for two pounds a week, that means 1000 calories a day. Here are some suggestions to help you start designing your programme. Notice the plan doesn't have to be the same each day. You can vary it to suit your schedule.

Plan of action

Day 1: cut out 500 calories from food

Day 2: cut out 300 calories from food & burn 200 calories in exercise

Day 3: cut out 200 calories from food & burn 300 calories in exercise

Use any combination you want as long as the numbers add up to 500 calories/day. I'll give you calorie counts of many common foods in Appendix A, so you can work out what you're eating and what needs cutting. And you already know how to burn calories—remember Chapter 6? So here are a few examples to get you thinking.

Examples of ways to cut food calories

▼ eliminate french fries—save 270 calories

▼ substitute "light" ice-cream for full fat brands—save 170 calories

▼ have four cups of popcorn instead of crisps—save 220 calories

▼ order a regular hamburger, rather than a quarter-pounder—save 300 calories

Examples of exercise that burns 220 calories

▼ walking at 4 mph for 1 hour

▼ a half-hour aerobics class or exercise video

▼ walking up and down stairs for 20 minutes

▼ cycling at 5 mph for 45 minutes

What do you eat now?

Do you have any idea how many calories or how much fat you take in in one day? Most people don't. Chances are you are eating much more than you think. Researchers have found that people generally underestimate what they eat by 25%. Keeping food records is vital to weight loss. I know this for a fact. In my many years of following dieters, I found the people who kept account of their food intake not only lost weight faster but continued to maintain their goal weight. No kidding. Write it down and you will take it off.

When you write down on paper what you eat, you tune into the fact that you are eating. A lot of food enters your mouth without your even knowing it. This is true especially if we are emotional eaters. Remember the last time you finished off a packet of crisps? Did you enjoy each and every crisp? More likely, by the time you realized the packet was empty, you wondered who ate them all.

Keeping track of what you eat for even a few weeks helps, but it's best to continue doing it until you're well on your way to achieving your goal. It's helpful for many reasons. As I already mentioned, it shows you what you are eating in terms of calories. Also, once you learn that something has 900 calories, and you have to write that down in your chart, it often stops you from plunging into it. Not always, but sometimes. So, recording everything makes you conscious of what you really eat and it helps you plan your diet.

Something that record-keeping is NOT meant to do is to make you feel guilty. There is no place in dieting for feeling bad about yourself. If you eat a high-fat food because you can't stop the craving, write it in your records, but don't be cross with yourself. Write it down with the calories so you can go back later and rethink that situation or that choice. Maybe in the future you can plan a different strategy so you won't be as tempted by that particular food.

Now that you see the point of food records, here are the details. First, make extra copies of the chart at the back to use throughout your programme. Then write down everything you eat and drink for one full week. I mean put down EVERY crumb, bite and nibble that enters your mouth. Be sure to guess the amount too. The first week is easy because all you enter is the food. Don't bother with calories yet. And, by all means, don't evaluate your diet as good or bad. Pretend you are a reporter whose only job is to take down the facts.

After the week has passed, take your chart and, using the food lists in Appendix A, figure out the calories for each food. This doesn't take as long as you think because, as you will see, you repeat a lot of foods. Most people eat only 20 different foods a week. It shows what creatures of habit we really are. Use the space below to record your favourites.

You may also find calorie information and bags of many of the foods you eat. Watc. serving sizes marked on packages. Start rea For example, a small packet of crisps is 300 ca can also get calorie information from many restaurants. Be bold and ask.

My twenty favourite foods

Food   Calories

1. _____

2. _____

3. _____

4. _____

5. _____

6. _____

7. _____

8. _____

9. _____

10. _____

11. _____

12._____

13._____

14._____

15._____

16._____

17._____

18._____

19._____

20._____

GETTING RID OF FAT PROMOTERS

There's no doubt about it—many foods we like put inches on our thighs. Do you recognize some of the worst offenders: fried foods, fast foods, crisps, nuts, pastries, butter, mayonnaise, salad dressings, and cheese? Go over your weekly diet record and circle the high-fat foods. Do you eat them every day or several times a day? How many calories do they each contain?

Add up your daily calories from your weekly food record. Are you shocked at the number? Can you see what to cut down on? Think about the foods you listed above. How much do you like them? Which ones don't you especially care about? Are there any you could easily give up or replace? Some you may eat out of habit or availability, not because you have strong feelings for them. Write these foods down.

Foods I can easily give up

Food   Calories

1. _____

2. _____

3. _____

4. _____

5. _____

6. _____

7. _____

8. _____

9. _____

10. _____

Now, what can you have instead that will also satisfy you? If you eat crisps at night when you watch TV and you decided you could live without them, what are you going to eat during the programmes? How about popcorn, fresh fruit, or an ice lolly? On the next page, write down what you plan to eat in place of these other foods, and how many calories will be saved by your choices.

The next chart shows favourite fat-makers and possible leaner alternatives. Look again at your list of favourite foods. What foods do you know for sure you can live without? What do you think would be likely replacements? Write these down also, with the calories you save, on the two charts that follow.

Better choices to help trim calories

Food	Calories	Food	Calories
Instead of...		Try...	
Big Mac	486	Regular hamburger	244
Large fries	533	Regular fries	267
Chocolate milkshake	360	Milk (semi-skimmed)	260 a pint
1 cup whole milk	150	1 cup non-fat milk	85
Taco Bell beef burrito	466	Taco Bell beef tostada	277
Club sandwich	590	Tuna sandwich	278
Steak (100 g)	350	Chicken (100 g)	175
Large ice-cream cone	340	Small ice-cream cone	120
Croissant	350	2 slices bread	150

Better choices for my diet

Food	Calories	Savings

Once you have decided on a few easy changes, like choosing a roast beef sandwich for lunch instead of a double whopper hamburger, practise doing this for a few weeks. Don't try to rearrange your whole life at once. Some people get excited and want instant results. Remember, permanent weight loss is a skill that takes time to learn.

When you feel the new changes you have made are not so difficult, go on to the next step. Again, go over your weekly food records and look for other foods that are high in fat calories. Maybe you are not ready to give some of these up—but what if you just ate LESS of these favourites? For example, do you have chocolates five days a week? How about having them three days a week? Do you have a chocolate milkshake once a day? How about cutting that down to every other day? Do you think that could work? It's another way to reduce those extra calories.

Things I could eat less of

Food	Calories	Savings

What about eating at home? Where can you cut here and still feel satisfied? Start with breakfast: do you like cereal? What kind of milk do you put on it? You could save up to 100 calories by changing from whole milk to low- or non-fat milk. Do you let your toast swim in butter? Could you use half the amount, or how about just jam? Butter is 100 calories a tablespoon and jam is 50 calories for the same amount. Peanut butter is the same as butter, so if you use both, double trouble. For lunch, do you make your sandwiches? How much mayonnaise do you use? The calories are almost as much as butter. Light mayo, mustard, and ketchup are at least half the calories. Check the numbers on condiments in the back of the book. Those tablespoons we add to a sandwich can lead to mega-calories.

Dinner is probably the most unpredictable. Some nights Mum cooks, sometimes Dad, maybe you go out to a restaurant or bring home take-away food. When another person in the family prepares the meal, it's hard to resist, usually because it all tastes so good. But if you are getting a lot of fried foods, sauces, and sweet food, you might make a suggestion that some evenings you have low calorie meals. I'm sure your parents would like to help you with your weight loss also, so why don't you educate them on calories? This may not be possible, I know. The family has learned to expect certain meals, and to upset the other members may not be worth it. If you know a food is very high in calories, rather than feel left out, just take a smaller portion. You are still cutting down.

Things to change when eating at home

Food	Calories	Savings

There are many ways to trim calories. In the chart below, I've listed some substitutes you may not have thought about yet.

SNACK ATTACKS

Ways to Reduce Fat Intake

Instead of ...   **Try ...**

Whole milk or cream   Non-fat
Sour cream, mayonnaise   Low- or non-fat yogurt
Cheese   Low-fat cheese
Ice-cream   Low-fat desserts
Regular mayonnaise   Light mayonnaise
Regular salad dressing   Yogurt and mayo blend
Fatty meats (prime rib)   Lean meats (flank steak)
Minced beef   Minced turkey
Beef   Chicken
Poultry with skin   Poultry without skin
Dark meat   Light meat
Meat or fish   Meat or fish
  (fried, breaded)   (poached, steamed)

Cream sauces	Spaghetti sauce
Crisps	Popcorn
Doughnut, pastry	Whole grain bread, bagel, muffin
Chocolate chip cookies	Crackers, ginger snaps
Butter on toast	Jam on toast
Fried foods	Poached, baked, or grilled foods

How about your snacks? They can really set you back. Yes, the calories are usually right up there, but worse, I think, is controlling the amount. Nobody eats one piece of chocolate, two biscuits, or five crisps. Snacking seems to send us into never-never land and before we know it, we eat the whole thing. Has this ever happened to you? It probably will again. Don't give up. You can learn to control your snacking so it doesn't sabotage your diet.

Think about the times you go crazy. What usually triggers it? Do you snack at the same time of the day, in the same place, and for the same reasons? Chances are you do. Many teenagers eat everything they can find right after school, others raid the refrigerator late at night, and some pig out when they're with friends. Think for a minute. What's your worst time with food?

Overeating is often tied to emotions. Generally speaking, overweight people tend to substitute food for feelings. We all do this to some extent. If we are angry, upset or even happy, we turn to food as our all-purpose soother. This is neither good nor bad. It is just an inappropriate response to an emotion, and it can be changed.

Working out what triggers you to overeat requires a little work and, once more, another list. Just knowing why you eat doesn't solve the problem. That takes time and practice. But it is a good start. Here are some examples to get you thinking.

What makes me overeat?

▼ I'm bored in the afternoon

▼ My mum or dad yells at me

▼ I fight with my sister or friends

▼ School homework is too hard

▼ It makes me feel good

▼ There are a lot of goodies in the house

▼ I have a bad day or I'm stressed

▼ My friends eat and don't gain weight

▼ Life's not fair

▼ No one understands me

Now write your own list below:

▼ _____
▼ _____
▼ _____
▼ _____
▼ _____

You probably aren't going to come up with all your reasons in one day. When they will come to mind is when you're diving into the last of the ice-cream. Like all the lists that you worked on earlier in the book, this one can be added to and altered as your life changes.

So now you have some idea of why you snack. It's great to know what's wrong, but if we don't have a solution to fix it, the information is useless. Some problems I can't help you with. If you have an unhappy home situation, you need to talk to someone who can help you. However, if the reason you snack uncontrollably is from boredom, loneliness, anger, or frustration, I may be able to give you some suggestions.

This time I want you to think of things you like to do. Remember your goal board? Maybe you can get ideas from there. List at least ten activities that you enjoy or would like to learn. When you are tempted by biscuits, cakes, and ice-cream, what else could you do that you would enjoy doing just as much? You don't want to wait until the chocolate is calling you. You need a plan in advance.

If you know you are likely to be bored tomorrow afternoon, think of something you can start before the boredom hits. But sometimes you don't know you are going to be cross or feel unloved. Then it is even more important to have some ideas for things that could make you feel better. Need some suggestions? How about: calling a friend, listening to music, dancing, playing tennis, walking the dog, getting a video, doing a jigsaw together, playing a game, reading a magazine or book, taking a bubble bath, going to a film, window shopping, riding your bike, cleaning your room, or planning a trip? Now it's your turn:

Things I Like To Do

1. _____

_____

2. _____

_____

3. _____

4. _____

5. _____

6. _____

7. _____

8. _____

9. _____

10. _____

When you snack, it is probably more important to control your overeating than it is to count each and every calorie; however, calories are important. So, if you are seriously watching those numbers, look at the chart below for some snacks that are under 100 calories.

Healthy Eating Keeps You Slim

I know I said I wouldn't try to change your eating habits too much, but as a mother and nutritionist, I just can't help putting in a plug for healthy food. In my experience most teenagers don't go out of their way to find nutritious food. My own daughter only eats beige foods (nothing green or yellow). I know I can't get you to eat carrots instead of fries, but how about giving some fresh fruits and vegetables a chance? They have few calories. If you like quantity eating, you can eat as much as you like of them. You may find out you like them.

Snacks under 100 calories

Food	Calories
Apple (1 medium)	90
Orange (1 medium)	75
Banana (1 small)	100
Grapes (20)	50
Watermelon (½ inch slice)	60
Carrot (1)	30
Baked potato (1 small)	100
Yogurt (4 oz)	60
Chocolate chip cookie (1)	100
Bagel (½)	80
Whole wheat bread (1 slice)	75
Egg, boiled (1)	90
Popcorn (normal carton)	25

You now know that fat makes you fat. Not only does it have the most calories, but it is also stored faster than other foods. Keep your eye on the fried foods (chicken, fish, crisps, potatoes)—they are the real killers. Literally. Fat has been linked with many adult diseases such as heart failure and high blood pressure. Stay healthy and limit the fat.

To be healthy, it is a good idea to eat a variety of foods every day. You should eat the following foods every day for your growing bodies. Check yourself and see how close you get to the goal.

For a balanced diet

Food Group	Minimum Daily Number of Servings
Meats or alternatives (beans, rice, dairy)	2
Milk & dairy products	4
Breads, cereals, pasta, rice	6
Vegetables	4
Fruits	2

Selecting foods from the different groups listed above ensures that you are getting all the nutrients you need to keep your body healthy. Eliminating even one food group from your diet means that you are missing some important vitamins and minerals. Over time, this lack of vitamins and minerals may cause unhealthy symptoms and even sickness.

FINE-TUNING YOUR PLAN

Have you filled out all the lists? If not, please go back and do it. It is so important to take the time to look at yourself, your feelings about losing weight, and your daily habits. Once you have, you are ready to plan the rest of your life. But let's just start with one day at a time!

Change doesn't happen in just one day or one month—even when you are highly motivated. Always make the easiest changes first. If you are not ready to exercise yet, start with reducing the calories. Or maybe it's easier for you to exercise than limit your food. That's fine too.

Think about your schedule for tomorrow. What are you doing? Where will you be when you eat? Who will you be eating with? Do you know any specific times of the day that might be particularly difficult? Will you be tempted to overeat? Think about all of these things before you sit down and write out your food choices.

Based on your past habits and favourite foods, what have you been eating for breakfast? Is that what you want tomorrow? Remember, you are either going to cut down your calories by 500, burn them through exercise, or do a combination of both. What will it be? In the morning, are you going to change your breakfast at all? Will it be different in terms of a substitution, or have you decided to use skimmed milk on your cornflakes rather than full fat milk, or stick to just marmalade on your toast, rather than butter and marmalade? Do you normally have a snack mid-morning? What will that be? How about lunch? Snack after school? Dinner? Write your plan down on a piece of paper you can carry with you and look at it during the day. Planning your day in advance will keep you focused on your goal and make it easier to follow through.

When you are making tomorrow's plan, look at the list of foods you can easily change. What did you write down as an alternative to that food? Reread your list of alternatives so you'll remember it. Don't let yourself get stuck without a plan of action. Be in control of your day. And, one more thing, if you haven't made a goal board or a list of thoughts for the day to take with you, go back to Chapter 5 and get busy. It will make the calorie counting much easier.

Above all, allow yourself time to alter your habits. And if you can't resist a fat-filled goody, it's OK. You are working at a skill and every day won't be perfect. The longer you keep at it, the easier it gets. Take it slowly. Forgive yourself for setbacks and you will succeed.

8
Eating Out, Tips for Success

Going to a restaurant can be a nightmare when you are trying to watch your calories. There are so many unknowns. You really can't expect to lose weight and keep it off unless you can learn what to order. At the start of the book I promised you could do this diet and still have some fun. So here are my rules for eating out. Remember: it is up to you to decide what foods are worth the calories, but when you eat out, keep these rules in mind:

Rule 1: Order only what you really want

Rule 2: Leave what you don't want

Rule 3: Take home what you can't eat

Rule 4: Share meals

Rule 5: Ask how it's cooked

The following chart lists many foods and ways of preparing them that you would commonly order in restaurants. In the left-hand column are foods which are high in fat and calories and therefore should generally be avoided. In the right-hand column are healthier, lower calorie alternatives which are just as satisfying.

Restaurant food guide

Usually not OK | *Usually OK*

Side Dishes/Starters

Usually not OK	Usually OK
Bread with butter, cheese, oil	Dry toast
Dips	Vegetable plate
Cream soups	Broth soups
Chef salad	Vegetable salad/sliced tomatoes
Salads with mayonnaise (eg potato)	Salads with no dressing
Stuffed Nan	Plain Nan
Papadoms (fried)	Papadoms (roasted)
Crisps	Plain tortillas

Meats

Usually not OK	Usually OK
Fried	Stir-fried, roasted
Deep-fried	Grilled, marinated
Baked in gravy or sauce	Baked
Cooked in butter sauce	Poached
Breaded	Barbecued
Dipped in batter	Grilled
Bhaji	Tandoori
Sausage/fatty meat	Lean meats, skinned chicken or fish

Potatoes

Usually not OK	Usually OK
With butter	Baked with sour cream and chives
Chips/potato skins	Boiled
Dauphinois	Roast

Sauces/dressings

Creamy white sauce	Peppers and mushrooms
Carbonara sauce	Tomato sauce
Pesto sauce	Marinara sauce
Bolognese	Napoletana
Sweet and sour sauce	Light wine sauce
Regular salad dressing	Low calorie salad dressing
Tartar sauce	Ketchup
Cheese sauce	Mustard
Croutons	Steak sauce

Desserts

Pastry/cake	Fresh fruit
Ice-cream	Frozen yogurt/sorbet
Chocolate	Mint

SURVIVING FAST-FOOD JOINTS

The bottom line on losing weight is to cut down on fats in the foods you eat most often. When you lower fat content you also lower the total number of calories. This does not mean, however, that you necessarily have to eat less food. Many people think that to diet means to starve—If they are not famished while dieting, they must be doing something wrong. It doesn't have to be like that. You can eat even more food if you are watching calories.

Fast-food restaurants are notorious for their high-fat foods, but since you will probably continue going to them, let me give you a few survival tactics. I am happy to say there are many more choices than there used to be, and I'm sure the future will bring us even more variety.

Low calorie choices

▼ Try not to use mayonnaise—ketchup or mustard is better. This will save you about 150 calories.

▼ Stay away from anything fried: fish, fries, onion rings, and chicken nuggets. They are packed with fat calories.

▼ Choose bread rather than a croissant.

▼ Try some of the low calorie salad dressings on green salad and avoid any salads—like potato, pasta and coleslaw—that are made with mayonnaise.

▼ One serving of nachos has twice the calories of a bean burrito.

▼ When ordering a pizza topping, remember that bacon has fewer calories than sausage or pepperoni. Have you ever tried pizza without cheese?

▼ Try a baked potato instead of fries. Sour cream is a better choice than butter.

▼ A chicken fajita is half the calories of a double beef burrito.

▼ You can have two scoops of a sorbet or non-fat yogurt for one scoop of deluxe ice-cream.

▼ Ask for a calorie chart, and make up your own mind.

Tips for success

You are all set to lose weight: you've designed your diet, exercise, and special circumstances. Here are some key points for making your plan a success.

- ▼ Start slowly. Most people want to lose 10 or 20 pounds in one week. This is not realistic. Permanent weight loss takes time. Look for no more than one or two pounds a week.

- ▼ Change one habit at a time. Even if you are gung-ho to turn your world upside down, forget it! Work on one meal or one snack only. When you feel comfortable with that, go on to another problem food or time.

- ▼ Always plan and write down your next day's eating schedule the night before. Be prepared for vulnerable times and determine how you are going to handle the situation.

- ▼ Eat regular meals. Don't go longer than five hours without eating. You will lose more weight this way even if you take in more calories.

- ▼ Drink two pints of water each day. That's eight eight-ounce glasses. If you are retaining water, drinking water helps to get rid of it.

- ▼ Diet with a friend if you can. It's good to have someone with whom you can share the experience. A support group is even better.

- ▼ Eat with friends. Some people don't want their friends to know they are dieting, so they avoid eating in public. Then when they get home, everything but the refrigerator goes in their mouth. Don't be embarrassed to watch what you eat with your friends, too.

- ▼ When you eat, do so without distractions. Don't watch TV or read. Pay attention to your food. Look at it, smell it, taste it, enjoy it.

- ▼ Eat slowly. It takes 20 minutes for your stomach to tell your brain you are full. If it helps, have an apple or something similar half an hour before dinner so you don't overeat.

- ▼ Keep problem foods out of the house and store up on lower-calorie snacks. You are more likely to resist temptation if it's not there.

- ▼ If you don't like something, don't eat it. Why waste your calories? (Be sensible though—this is not an excuse to stop eating fruit and vegetables and other essential food.)

- ▼ When you blow it, and you will, forgive yourself and go on. Weight loss is a process that you don't learn overnight.

- ▼ Record all you eat with the caloric value until you know what you are taking in. Do it for a minimum of four weeks. Three months is even better.

- ▼ Picture yourself as the person you know you can be!

Now you know it all. You have the guidelines to design your own *safe* diet plan. Just know that is is possible and know you are going to succeed. You are wonderful as you are right now. Soon, you will feel even more wonderful because you are doing something to make your life healthier. I wish you all success.

Appendix A
Calories in Common Foods

This list is just to give you an idea of the number of calories in common foods. There is nutritional information on the packaging of most food so you should be able to find out the number of calories in the food you most often eat.

The numbers given here are rounded off to the nearest 5 calories, and fast foods are in a separate section at the end.

*B*reads *(1 slice unless otherwise stated) and bread-like food*

Cream crackers	35
Breadsticks	40
Whole wheat, sliced thin	40
Dinner roll	60
Croutons (1 tbsp)	70
White	70
French	70
Crumpet	80
Hot dog bun	100
Hamburger bun	130
Muffin	130
Tortilla, flour	150
Pitta bread	150
Bagel	180
Croissant	190
Tostada shell	200

*C*akes and biscuits *(1 slice/biscuit)*

Jaffa cake	50
Plain digestive	50
Fruit and nut biscuit	60
Chocolate digestive	80
Chocolate cake, Sara Lee, fat-free	110
Fruit Club	120
Breakaway	125
Chocolate cup cake, Lyons	130
Almond slice, Mr Kipling	135
Apple pie, Lyons	200
Choux bun, St Michael	235

*C*ereal

Bran flakes (typical serving 30 g)	160
Shredded wheat (2 biscuits)	160
Cornflakes (typical 30 g serving)	160
Muesli (typical 60 g serving)	215
Alpen (typical 60 g) serving)	380

*C*heese *(100 g or 3.5 oz)*

Ricotta, light	80
Ricotta	140
Mozzarella, part-skimmed	250
Feta	260
String cheese	280
Camembert or Brie	315
Cream cheese	350
Swiss	385
Cheddar	418

*C*ondiments *(1 tbsp)*

Chilli sauce	3
Horseradish	4
Salsa	5
Taco sauce	6
Mustard, yellow	11
Worcestershire sauce	12
Ketchup	15
Coffee Mate	16
Cream, half and half	20
Mustard, Dijon	24
Sour cream	26
Brown sugar	35
Mayonnaise, reduced calorie	50
Cream cheese	50
Honey	65
Nutella	90
Butter	100
Margarine	100
Butter	100

*D*rinks *(non-alcoholic)*

Diet cola	0
Bitter lemon, Schweppes (100 ml)	10
Apple drink, Tango (100 ml)	10
Freshly squeezed orange juice, Tesco (100 ml)	40
Ribena (100 ml)	40
Lemonade (330 ml can)	75
Orangina (half pint)	110

*E*ggs *(1 unless otherwise stated)*

Egg white	20

Egg yolk	60
Boiled egg (size 2)	90
Quiche (quarter)	235
Cheese omelette (2 eggs, 30 g cheese, a tbsp butter)	295
Ham and cheese omelette	380
Spanish omelette (3 eggs)	425

*F*ish *(100 grams/3.5 oz, unless otherwise stated)*

White fish: sole, cod, halibut, snapper	
steamed	85
fried lightly	195
breaded & fried	245
Pale coloured fish: swordfish, tuna	
baked, grilled	160
fried	210
Dark coloured fish: salmon, mackerel	
baked, grilled	245
fried	290
Fish fingers (1)	
grilled	50
fried	60
Prawns, steamed	100
Smoked salmon	105
Rainbow trout, steamed	150
Sardines in oil, drained	210

*F*ruit

Apricot (medium)	15
Prune, dried (1 large)	20
Peach, medium	35
Tomato, medium	35

CALORIES IN COMMON FOODS

Grapefruit, half	40
Plum	45
Strawberries, 1 cup	45
Watermelon, 1 slice	50
Orange, medium	80
Pineapple (1 slice)	80
Apple (medium)	90
Banana (small)	90
Pear (medium)	90
Grapes (about 20)	100

Ice-cream/ice-lollies/yoghurt

Orange Maid (Lyons Maid)	45
Choc Ice (Lyons Maid)	130
Strawberry Cornetto (Wall's)	205
Choc and nut Cornetto (Wall's)	220
Mint choc chip Cornetto (Wall's)	235
Sainsbury's natural low fat yoghurt	110
Raspberry yoghurt (Ski)	150

Meat (100 g/3.5 oz – unless otherwise stated)

BEEF
Sirloin, lean	200
Sirloin, with fat	225
Flank steak, grilled	220
Mince, extra lean	225
Mince, lean	260
Chuck, blade, lean	210
Chuck, blade, with fat	285
Sainsbury's British beef sausage (1)	120

PORK
Pork chops, lean	195

Pork chops, with fat	230
Pork, sirloin roast, lean	210
Pork, sirloin roast, with fat	250
Ham, lean	210
Ham, with fat	290
Sainsbury's British premium pork sausage (1)	135

Bacon
streaky	330
other	280

*P*asta *(100 g/3.5 oz)*

Dried spaghetti,	135
Dried tagliatelle	135
Fresh spaghetti	140
Fresh Penne	140
Fresh tagliatelle	145
Tortelloni	165

*P*oultry *(100 g/3.5 oz)*

Chicken breast, meat only	165
Chicken breast, meat and skin	195
Chicken breast, meat and skin fried	260
Chicken, dark meat only	210
Chicken, dark meat and skin	245
Turkey breast, meat only	155
Duck (roasted)	335

*S*alads *(average helping)*

Carrot and raisin	80
Fresh fruit	90

Bean	110
Fettuccini with vegetable	110
Potato with yogurt dressing	120
Coleslaw	150
Rice	150
Waldorf	150
Potato with mayonnaise	170

Sweets and snacks

SAVOURY

Apricot date bar (30 g bar)	85
Cheddars, McVities (1 biscuit)	89
Walkers crisps (28 g pack)	149
Hula hoops (30 g packet)	155
Real McCoy crisps (40 g packet)	211

SWEET

Chewing gum (1 stick)	10
Fruit pastilles (1)	10
Fox's Glacier mint (1)	15
Munchies (1)	25
After Eight (1)	65
Flake 99	65
Chocolate buttons (1 packet)	175
M&Ms, plain (1 packet)	240
Caramel bar	245
KitKat (four fingers)	250
Mars bar	280

Soups

Vegetable and beef Batchelor's cup-a-soup (24 g dried sachet)	90
Oxtail, Crosse & Blackwell, 283 g tin	100

Tomato soup, Campbell's, 295 g tin	180
Cream of leek, Baxters (425 g can)	220
Cream of mushrooms, Baxters (425 g can)	230
Cream of tomato, Baxters (425 g can)	300

*V*egetables and rice *(unless otherwise stated average helping)*

Lettuce	10
Celery	20
Courgette, fresh	20
Broccoli, fresh	40
Green beans, fresh	40
Carrots, fresh	45
Asparagus	50
Onion, fresh	60
Artichoke, medium	65
Peas, fresh	80
Corn on the cob	170
Heinz baked beans, small tin	205
Weightwatchers	115
Potato, medium	220
Potato, mashed with butter and whole milk	240
White long-grain rice	220
Brown long-grain rice	240
Fried rice	320

*F*ast food

BURGERS ETC

McDonald's hamburger	245
Burger King hamburger	255
McDonald's cheeseburger	300
Big Mac	485
McDonald's quarter pounder with cheese	500

CALORIES IN COMMON FOODS

Burger King Whopper — 540

McDonald's chicken nuggets (6) — 265
McDonald's fillet o' fish — 350
Sausage and egg Mcmuffin — 425
Burger King spicy beanburger — 545

FRENCH FRIES
McDonald's regular — 265
McDonald's medium — 380
McDonald's large — 535
Burger King regular — 290

PIZZA (2 slices, medium size)
Domino's cheese — 375
Pizza Hut thin 'n' crispy cheese — 400
Pizza Hut thin 'n' crispy pepperoni — 415
Domino's ham — 415
Domino's pepperoni — 460

SALADS
McDonald's garden salad — 110
McDonald's chef — 230
Taco Bell salad with shell — 940

MILKSHAKES
Burger King chocolate milkshake — 330
McDonald's chocolate milkshake — 365

DESSERTS
McDonald's apple pie — 220
McDonald's donut (plain) — 285
Burger King apple pie — 320

I LOOKED IN THE MIRROR AND SCREAMED

*F*OOD RECORD AND CALORIE LOG

Write down the foods you eat under each meal heading. Record the calories und
"Out". By subtracting Calories "Out" from Calories "In" you get your net calorie

MONDAY	Calories "In"	TUESDAY	Calories "In"	WEDNESDAY	Calories "In"	THU
Breakfast		Breakfast		Breakfast		Brea
Snack		Snack		Snack		Sna
Lunch		Lunch		Lunch		Lun
Snack		Snack		Snack		Sna
Dinner		Dinner		Dinner		Din
Snack		Snack		Snack		Sna
Total Calories "In" (**A**)		Total Calories "In" (**A**)		Total Calories "In" (**A**)		Tota Calc "In"
EXERCISE	Calories "Out"(**B**)	EXERCISE	Calories "Out"(**B**)	EXERCISE	Calories "Out"(**B**)	EXE
Net Calories (**A–B**)		Net Calories (**A–B**)		Net Calories (**A–B**)		Net (**A–**

GOALS FOR NEXT WEEK

_____   _____

_____   _____

_____   _____

CALORIES IN COMMON FOOD

Week	From	To

es "In". Write your exercise for the day, and record the calories it burns under **Calories** r the day.

Calories "In"		Calories "In"		Calories "In"		Calories "In"
	FRIDAY Breakfast		**SATURDAY** Breakfast		**SUNDAY** Breakfast	
	Snack		Snack		Snack	
	Lunch		Lunch		Lunch	
	Snack		Snack		Snack	
	Dinner		Dinner		Dinner	
	Snack		Snack		Snack	
	Total Calories "In" (**A**)		Total Calories "In" (**A**)		Total Calories "In" (**A**)	
Calories "Out"(**B**)	EXERCISE	Calories "Out"(**B**)	EXERCISE	Calories "Out"(**B**)	EXERCISE	Calories "Out"(**B**)
	Net Calories (**A–B**)		Net Calories (**A–B**)		Net Calories (**A–B**)	

Total Calories for the week:

Appendix B
Resources: Where to Get More Help

BOOKS

EATING YOUR HEART OUT
Buckroyd (Optima, 1994, £6.99)
This book discusses the emotional traumas which can cause eating disorders including obsessional dieting, compulsive eating, bingeing and vomiting or anorexia.

BULIMIA NERVOSA
Cooper (Robinson Publishing, 1993, £5.99)
This is full of information about bulimia nervosa, written in clear, easy-to-understand language. The first part deals with its physical and psychological effects, the second gives the reader a practical way of tackling the problem.

CATHERINE
Dunbar (Penguin, 1986, £4.99)
This is Maureen Dunbar's moving account of her daughter's 7-year battle against Anorexia Nervosa – which she ultimately lost.

NEVER DIET AGAIN
Kano (Thorsons, 1990, £5.99)
This book helps you break free from weight/dieting obsessions.

TALKING ABOUT ANOREXIA – How to Cope with Life without Starving
Monro (Sheldon, £4.99)

This is written by a recovered anorexic who also worked as an agony aunt. This is particularly recommended for teenagers.

HELP FOR EATING DISORDERS

Eating Disorders Association (EDA)
Sackville Place
44 Magdalen Street
Norwich
Norfolk NR3 1JU

Youth helpline: (0603) 765050 Open 4–6 pm, Mon-Wed
General helpline (0603) 621414

All the above books (and others) are available through the EDA (send cheque plus £0.80 for p&p). The EDA can also provide information on groups local to you, dealing with eating disorders.

Other books published by Piccadilly Press for teenagers

Non-fiction

STAYING COOL, SURVIVING SCHOOL:
  Secondary School Strategies
by Rosie Rushton

"A light-hearted but useful sprint through some pitfalls of secondary school . . . will cheer you up."
  Scotland on Sunday

THIRTEENSOMETHING:
  A Survivor's Guide
by Jane Goldman

"... a witty, light-hearted guide for young teenagers."
  Daily Mail

DON'T PICK ON ME:
  How to Handle Bullying
by Rosemary Stones

"At last someone has written clear and welcome advice for children on how to handle the widespread problem of bullying."
  Daily Mail

SEX: HOW? WHY? WHAT?
  The Teenager's Guide
by Jane Goldman

"One of the best books I've seen on the subject."
  Woman's Weekly

STYLE BLITZ:
   Grooming and Good Looks for Boys
by Helen Thorne

"Helen Thorne has written the essential young male guide to making the best of yourself."
   Daily Express

YOU'RE MY BEST FRIEND – I HATE YOU!
   Friends – Getting, Losing and Keeping Them
by Rosie Rushton

"...brilliant new book..."
   Shout Magazine

Coming soon:

IT'S NOT YOUR FAULT:
   How to Handle Your Parents' Divorce
by Rosemary Stones

It's always difficult when parents divorce, but it's an awful lot worse when you don't know what is happening or what to expect. This book prepares children for the practical and emotional impact of parents' divorce.

DON'T BLAME ME – I'M A GEMINI!
   Astrology for Teenagers
by Reina James Reinstein and Mike Reinstein

Find out the personality traits associated with your Sun sign, how you get on with family, friends, teachers, the opposite sex, and much more in this wonderfully entertaining book.

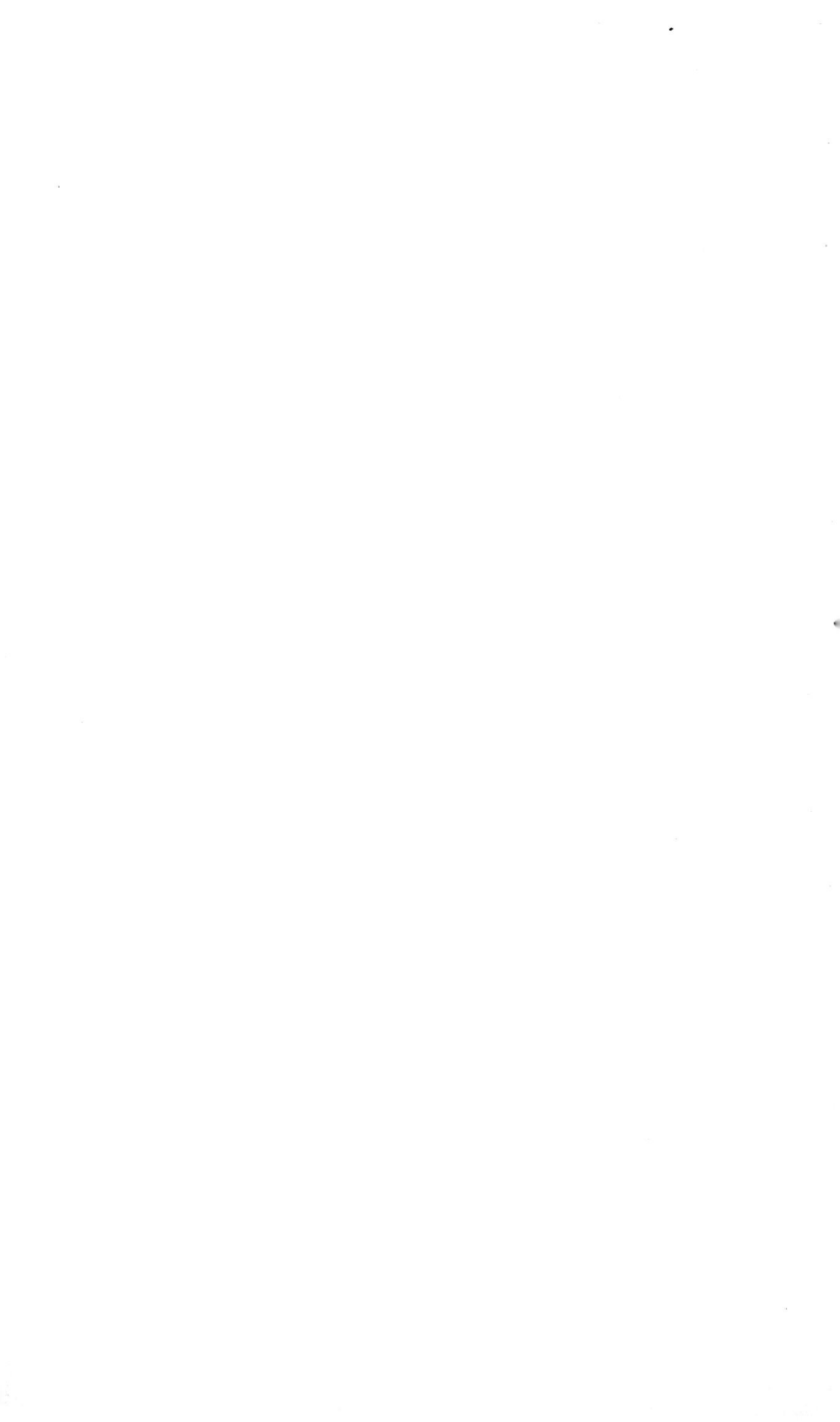